Passing the Certified Bariatric Nurses Exam

Andrew Loveitt
Margaret M. Martin • Marc A. Neff
Editors

Passing the Certified Bariatric Nurses Exam

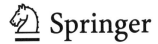 Springer

Editors
Andrew Loveitt
Rowan University
Stratford, NJ
USA

Marc A. Neff
Kennedy Univ. Hospital - Cherry Hill
Center for Surgical Weight Loss
Cherry Hill, NJ
USA

Margaret M. Martin, BSN, RN, CBN
Kennedy University Hospital
Stratford, NJ
USA

ISBN 978-3-319-41702-8   ISBN 978-3-319-41703-5   (eBook)
DOI 10.1007/978-3-319-41703-5

Library of Congress Control Number: 2016962446

Printed on acid-free paper

This Springer imprint is published by Springer Nature
The registered company is Springer International Publishing AG
The registered company address is: Gewerbestrasse 11, 6330 Cham, Switzerland

To my wife, Courtenay, for all you do
Andrew Loveitt

My 3 children...Jamie, Andrew, and Dylan
Marc A. Neff

My 3 children...Matthew, David, and Claire
Margaret M. Martin

Preface

I have been a caring for bariatric surgery patients since 1999. From the beginning, I realized that this is a different patient population. As different as caring for the elderly, the pregnant patient, the pediatric patient, the health-care professional has to take into account a different physiology and group of disease processes that can manifest themselves differently. A bariatric patient could have a complication, a GI leak, but have minimal findings on physical exam or go into respiratory arrest postop as the general anesthetic slowly diffuses out of their adipose tissue. The knowledge that this patient population is unique is vital to good outcomes and proper patient care.

The ASMBS recognized the need for specialized nursing in 2006 and created an exam to help credential those nurses best suited to care for the bariatric patient. The Certified Bariatric Nurse Exam credentials a nurse for 4 years that they have mastered the expertise necessary to care for this patient population. According to the ASMBS website, a nurse qualifies to take the exam if they are:

> A currently licensed professional nurse (RN or equivalent for international nurses) with a valid license number or equivalent, and have been a professional nurse for a minimum of 2 years. And they have worked with morbidly obese and bariatric surgery patients for a minimum of 24 months in the preceding four years, predominately in the Bariatric surgery process. (i.e.: pre-operative, peri-operative or post-operative/follow-up care).

The CBN Examination consists of 170 multiple-choice items. The test presents each question with four response alternatives (A, B, C, and D). One of these represents the single best response, and credit is granted only for selection of this response. Candidates are allowed three hours (180 min) to complete this test.

But more so than these qualifications and this test is a profound understanding of what a bariatric patient is and what the surgery means to them. Obesity is the only remaining acceptable form of discrimination. An individual in this country may not be discriminated against based on their age, their gender, their race, their religious convictions, or their sexual orientation. However, the obese patient is often thought of as sloppy, depressed, ashamed, lazy, and socially dysfunctional. They progress more slowly in their careers. But, as a surgeon, I will tell you that there is no more satisfying patient population to care for. They appreciate that someone is giving them the attention they need, offering them an opportunity to be healthier, to live life, to no longer be trapped inside their body, and to do the things that many of us take for granted, from sitting in a booth at a restaurant, to flying on a plane without a seat extender, to bending over and tying their shoes without feeling like their head is going to explode. When patients come back to my office having changed the direction of their lives, I feel like I have truly made a difference. Patients forget who did their appendectomy, but they will never forget who did their bariatric surgery and who took care of them before and after that life-changing event.

I am blessed that at my institution to have four certified bariatric nurses. They participate in patient care, preoperatively and postoperatively. They facilitate the patient experience from teaching the preoperative class to running the support groups. I don't think that care and compassion of the bariatric patient requires this exam or a certificate to be hung on the wall. I do however agree that efficient and appropriate care demands a level of competency that this exam tests for. It is for that purpose that this book was created.

Cherry Hill, NJ, USA   Marc A. Neff, MD, FACS, FASMBS

Contents

1   Introduction to Passing the Certified Bariatric Nurse Exam   1
    Andrew Loveitt

2   Introduction to Bariatric Surgery   3
    Marc A. Neff

3   The History of Metabolic Surgery   7
    Wiliam Stembridge

4   The Obesity Epidemic 11
    Eve Bruneau

5   Indications for Bariatric Surgery 15
    Eve Bruneau

6   Basic Anatomy and Physiology of the Gastrointestinal Tract 19
    Eve Bruneau

7   Medical Strategies for Weight Loss 27
    Andrew Loveitt

8   Restrictive Versus Malabsorptive Procedures
    in Bariatric Surgery 33
    William Stembridge

9   Preoperative Evaluation of the Bariatric Surgery Patient 37
    William Stembridge

10 Positioning the Bariatric Patient in the OR 45
    Neha Patel and Elton Taylor

11 Anesthesia in the Bariatric Patient 51
    Sunny Kar

12 General Overview of the Laparoscopic Adjustable Band 55
    Nidhi Khanna

13 Laparoscopic Gastric Band: Early and Late Complications 57
    Nidhi Khanna

14   **Laparoscopic Gastric Band: Pros and Cons**.   61
     Nidhi Khanna

15   **General Overview of the Laparoscopic Sleeve Gastrectomy**   65
     Andrew Loveitt

16   **Laparoscopic Sleeve Gastrectomy: Pros and Cons**   67
     Andrew Loveitt

17   **Laparoscopic Sleeve Gastrectomy: The Procedure**   73
     Andrew Loveitt

18   **Laparoscopic Sleeve Gastrectomy: Recognizing and Treating
     Complications**   79
     Andrew Loveitt

19   **General Overview of the Laparoscopic Roux-en-Y
     Gastric Bypass**.   85
     Roshin Thomas

20   **Laparoscopic Roux-en-Y Gastric Bypass: The Procedure**   87
     Roshin Thomas

21   **Roux-en-Y Gastric Bypass: Pros and Cons**   91
     Roshin Thomas

22   **Roux-en-Y Gastric Bypass: Recognizing and Treating
     Complications**   95
     Roshin Thomas

23   **Biliopancreatic Diversion with Duodenal Switch (BPD/DS)**. 101
     Marc A. Neff

24   **Special Equipment for the Bariatric Patient** 105
     Lisa Harasymczuk

25   **Complications of Bariatric Surgery: Gastrointestinal Leak**. 111
     Tatyana Faynberg

26   **Complications of Bariatric Surgery: Venous Thromboembolism** . . . 115
     Tatyana Faynberg

27   **Complications of Bariatric Surgery: Obstruction** 119
     Tatyana Faynberg

28   **Complications of Bariatric Surgery: Dehydration** 123
     Lynn J. Stott

29   **Nasogastric Tube Placement in the Bariatric Patient** 127
     Rahul Sharma

30 Pharmacologic Considerations in Obesity 131
Mara Piltin

31 Basic Nutrition in Obese Patients 135
Alyssa Luning and Cheri Leahy

32 Pre- and Postoperative Nutrition Evaluations 147
Alyssa Luning, Cheri Leahy, and Lisa Harasymczuk

33 Follow-Up and Dietary Progression After Bariatric Surgery 153
Nidhi Khanna, Cheri Leahy, and Alyssa Luning

Additional Review Questions 157

Contributors

Eve Bruneau, DO Department of General Surgery, Rowan University, Stratford, NJ, USA

Tatyana Faynberg, DO Department of General Surgery, Rowan University, Stratford, NJ, USA

Lisa Harasymczuk, DO Department of General Surgery, Rowan University, Stratford, NJ, USA

Sunny Kar, DO Department of General Surgery, Rowan University, Stratford, NJ, USA

Nidhi Khanna, DO Department of General Surgery, Rowan University, Stratford, NJ, USA

Cheri Leahy, RDN Kennedy Health Alliance, Cherry Hill, NJ, USA

Andrew Loveitt, DO Department of General Surgery, Rowan University, Stratford, NJ, USA

Alyssa Luning, RDN Kennedy Health Alliance, Cherry Hill, NJ, USA

Marc A. Neff, MD, FACS, FASMBS General Surgery, Kennedy Health Alliance, Cherry Hill, NJ, USA

Neha Patel, DO Department of General Surgery, Rowan University, Stratford, NJ, USA

Mara Piltin, DO Department of General Surgery, Rowan University, Stratford, NJ, USA

Rahul Sharma, DO, MPH Department of General Surgery, Rowan University, Stratford, NJ, USA

Wiliam Stembridge, DO Department of General Surgery, Rowan University, Stratford, NJ, USA

Lynn J. Stott, RN, CMSRN, CBN Kennedy University Hospital, Stratford, NJ, USA

Elton Taylor, DO, MBA Department of General Surgery, Rowan University, Stratford, NJ, USA

Roshin Thomas, DO Department of General Surgery, Rowan University, Stratford, NJ, USA

Introduction to Passing the Certified Bariatric Nurse Exam

Andrew Loveitt

Obesity is an epidemic in the United States of America. This may not be news to most but even the experienced healthcare practitioner must find the following statistics startling:

- 34.9 % or 78.9 million US adults are obese (BMI greater than 30) [1].
- The annual medical cost of obesity in the United States was estimated to be $147 billion in 2008 [2].
- Obesity is associated with nearly one in five US deaths [3].

The fight against obesity became prevalent in 1999 when the US Centers for Disease Control and Prevention (CDC) first published state-based maps making the rapid progression of obesity across our nation obvious to even the most casual observer (http://www.cdc.gov/obesity/data/prevalence-maps.html). The fight has continued to rage and sadly we are losing the battle.

This is not for lack of effort. 2013 marked an important year as the American Medical Association officially declared obesity a disease in an effort to open up new resources for patients and those trying desperately to help them. The United States continues to spend trillions of dollars along with uncountable man-hours to fight this epidemic. Despite this enormous public health effort, national rates of obesity are still at an all-time high [1]. What can be done?

Enter the surgeon. While various forms of weight-loss surgery have been available for decades, there has been a recent boom in demand. This is partially a result of the increasing prevalence of the disease but other forces are in effect. The procedures being performed today, in a large part thanks to laparoscopy, have much lower complication rates than those years ago. Surgeons specializing in these techniques

A. Loveitt, DO
Department of General Surgery, Rowan University, Stratford, NJ, USA
e-mail: Loveitan@rowan.edu

© Springer International Publishing Switzerland 2017
A. Loveitt et al. (eds.), *Passing the Certified Bariatric Nurses Exam*,
DOI 10.1007/978-3-319-41703-5_1

have become prevalent. Perhaps most importantly the stigmata of undergoing a bariatric procedure are being lifted. This is not by accident but through a concerted effort by organizations such as the American Society of Bariatric Physicians and American Society for Metabolic and Bariatric Surgery (ASMBS).

Why are we writing this book? As bariatric surgery has become more prevalent, so has the demand on hospitals to meet the specialized needs of the bariatric patient. We have gained experience at our own bariatric facility which is accredited by the American College of Surgeons and have affirmed our belief that truly excellent care starts with excellent nursing. The certified bariatric nurse certification was developed by the ASMBS to establish a professional standard for qualified bariatric surgical nurses and validate a breadth of knowledge and skill necessary to care for the bariatric surgical patient. These specialized nurses are who we want caring for our patients and our patients feel the same way.

Of course with any certification comes a test and the CBN does not disappoint. The CBN exam can be taken by any RN who has worked with bariatric surgery patients for at least 24 months in the previous 4 years. It is administered at testing centers across the United States in February and July. Fees vary from $250 to $480. The test consists of 170 multiple-choice questions each with four answer choices. Test takers have 3 hours to complete the exam, and results are mailed 4–8 weeks after test day. The certification is good for 4 years after which recertification is necessary. For more information visit: https://asmbs.org/professional-education/cbn/cbn-certification-faq

Unfortunately there is a dearth of knowledge regarding what this test covers and how to practice for it. Word of mouth simply will not cut it! We have created *Passing the Certified Bariatric Nurse Exam* to aid you toward not only passing the test and advancing your career but, most importantly, providing more complete and up-to-date care to your patients.

The ASMBS website (listed above) does have excellent resources detailing what will be included on your test, and we suggest you review these materials before getting started with your exam preparation. We intend for this book to be used as a supplement along with other resources for the CBN test. The introductory paragraphs should provide sufficient background knowledge, and the review questions are meant to solidify it. Just before the exam, review the questions multiple times. This should help trigger your knowledge and also identify areas of weakness which will allow for more focused study.

Best of luck!

References

1. Ogden CL, Carroll MD, Kit BK, Flegal KM (2014) Prevalence of childhood and adult obesity in the United States 2011–2012. JAMA 311(8):806–814
2. Finkelstein EA, Trogdon JG, Cohen JW, Dietz W (2009) Annual medical spending attributable to obesity: payer-and service-specific estimates. Health Aff 28(5):822–831
3. Masters RK, Reither EN, Powers DA, Yang YC, Burger AE, Link BG (2012) The impact of obesity on US mortality levels: the importance of age and cohort factors in population estimates. Am J Public Health 103(10):1895–1901

Introduction to Bariatric Surgery

2

Marc A. Neff

Weight loss surgery (WLS) has come a long way since its early introduction. It currently is safer than heart operations, safer than hip operations, and carries a mortality rate no more than a regular laparoscopic cholecystectomy. This is because of dedicated bariatric and minimally invasive surgical training programs, supervision by the American College of Surgeons (ACS) and the American Society for Metabolic and Bariatric Surgery (ASMBS), and the training of Certified Bariatric Nurses (CBN).

In addition to the improvement in the safety profile of the surgical procedures, so has our understanding of the nature of obesity. It is now implicated in over 65 different medical conditions ranging from sleep apnea to diabetes, from hypertension to hyperlipidemia. In addition, obesity has been found to be a contributing risk in over 11 different malignancies, including breast and colon cancer.

The surgical procedures work in a variety of ways. Some procedures, such as the lap band and gastric balloon, are restrictive in nature. They work by restricting a patient's eating habits. Other procedures combine a malabsorptive element, such as the gastric bypass and duodenal switch. Still others work with combination of restrictive and hormonal mechanisms, such as the gastric sleeve. Regardless of the surgical procedure chosen, they are all functional tools to facilitate weight loss given the proper follow-up, diet, exercise plan, and lifestyle modification.

All surgical procedures suffer from the risks of bleeding, infection, and reaction to anesthesia. These can be successfully treated with proper identification and early intervention and still lead to successful weight loss. Even a leak can be treated successfully, in a minimally invasive fashion, if recognized early. The leading cause of death in all patients undergoing surgical weight loss is pulmonary embolism. This risk is a 1 in 250 chance, but 1 in 3 patients who suffer an embolism will not survive.

M.A. Neff, MD, FACS, FASMBS
General Surgery, Kennedy Health Alliance, Cherry Hill, NJ, USA
e-mail: M.Neff@kennedyhealth.org

© Springer International Publishing Switzerland 2017
A. Loveitt et al. (eds.), *Passing the Certified Bariatric Nurses Exam*,
DOI 10.1007/978-3-319-41703-5_2

3

Weight loss surgery is becoming increasingly popular. In 2016, nearly 200,000 procedures are expected to be performed. The numbers of patients in our country alone that have had WLS number in the millions. Every health care practitioner in their career, regardless of their field, is likely to encounter patients who have had weight loss surgery. It is important to understand the procedures performed, their mechanisms of action, the necessary follow-up, and the potential long-term complications.

Review Questions

1. Choose the correct statement. Weight loss surgery is:

   A. More dangerous than heart operations
   B. More dangerous than hip operations
   C. More dangerous than a laparoscopic cholecystectomy
   D. Safer because of specific training programs for both physicians and nurses and supervision by national organizations

2. Weight loss surgery (WLS) has been linked to:

   A. Infertility
   B. Endometrial cancers
   C. GERD
   D. Type II diabetes
   E. All of the above

3. All surgical procedures are a tool to help the patient achieve successful weight loss. Other important components are:

   A. Diet, exercise, lifestyle management
   B. The proper scale
   C. Having three protein shakes a day
   D. Cleansing once a month

4. The leading cause of death after weight loss surgery is:

   A. Myocardial infarction
   B. Sepsis
   C. Pulmonary embolism
   D. Post-op bleeding

Answers

1. The answer is *D*. The specific requirements for surgeon credentialing are laid out by the SAGES, SLS, ACS, and ASMBS organizations. In addition, data at credentialed centers is submitted for review by the ACS. The addition of the CBN has further improved patient safety.
2. The answer is *E*. WLS has impact on 65 different medical conditions with resolution rates ranging from 50 to 100%. The possibility of resolution of medical comorbidities such as type 2 diabetes depends on the

severity of the disease, the duration the patient has been in treatment, the type of surgery performed, and the degree of weight loss. Obesity has been implicated in 11 different malignancies related, in part, to changing estrogen levels, poor diet, and poor patient screening.

3. The answer is *A*. All procedures will change how quickly a patient eats, how much they eat, and the types of food they eat. But this is only part of the successful equation for surgical weight loss. A patient still needs to pay attention to their diet, follow up with a dietician, have regular blood work to check protein and vitamin levels, manage their stress, and exercise regularly. The postoperative follow-up is best individualized towards the patient's specific goals, tailored with regard to their progress, and lifelong. A fitness tracker and food log have been shown to increase total amount and duration of weight loss.

4. The answer is *C*. The leading cause of death is pulmonary embolism. This is characterized by the acute onset of shortness of breath, hypoxia, hypotension, chest pain, a sense of impending doom, and tachycardia. The best treatment is prevention. Patients should be ambulatory within 4 h of the surgical procedure, and patients at high risk (family or personal history of a PE, BMI over 60, or immobility) should be considered for prophylactic IVC filter. While the other causes may also be life-threatening, they are all very treatable with prompt identification.

The History of Metabolic Surgery

3

Wiliam Stembridge

Metabolic surgery and its offshoot bariatric surgery have been under development for decades with many rapid advances in recent years. The earliest operations performed for the express intent of weight loss were performed in the 1950s at the University of Minnesota. Dr. Richard Varco completed the first jejunoileal bypass in 1953, a procedure that involved bypassing the majority of the small bowel while leaving the stomach intact [1]. Patients enjoyed a high level of success in weight loss but were fraught with complications including severe vitamin deficiencies, gas-bloat syndrome, kidney stones, liver degeneration, and even mental status changes. The excluded portion of the intestine often suffered complications due to bacterial overgrowth, and a large majority of these patients have had their operations revised [2].

Dr. Edward Mason was trained at the University of Minnesota during the advent of metabolic surgery and later taught surgery at the University of Iowa. There, in 1966, he developed the first gastric bypass procedure consisting of a horizontal gastric division accompanied by a gastrojejunostomy. Inspiration arose from the weight loss observed in patients following gastric resections for peptic ulcers. The procedure was very successful and replaced the jejunoileal bypass in short order. In 1977 back at the University of Minnesota, Drs. John Alden and Ward Griffen advanced the gastric bypass to include gastric cross stapling and a Roux-en-Y reconstruction to publish what we now know as the classic Roux-en-Y gastric bypass. The first laparoscopic Roux-en-Y was performed in 1994 by Dr. Alan Wittgrove [1].

Various iterations of gastric banding, a purely restrictive procedure, have been used throughout the history of bariatric surgery beginning in the late 1970s. The vertical banded gastroplasty was originally devised as a safer alternative to the

W. Stembridge, DO (✉)
Department of General Surgery, Rowan University, Stratford, NJ, USA
e-mail: stembrwi@rowan.edu

© Springer International Publishing Switzerland 2017
A. Loveitt et al. (eds.), *Passing the Certified Bariatric Nurses Exam*,
DOI 10.1007/978-3-319-41703-5_3

Roux-en-Y gastric bypass. A number of materials have been used to segregate portions of the stomach including Marlex mesh, Dacron and PTFE vascular grafts, and ultimately silicone in most modern adjustable bands. The adjustable gastric band is still in use and prevalent in modern bariatric surgery [1].

A pair of similar operations, the duodenal switch and biliopancreatic diversion, is less common in modern practice as they require the highest level of surgical acumen and also carry the potential for serious complication. The more common sleeve gastrectomy is said to have originated as the more effective portion of a two-part duodenal switch. The sleeve gastrectomy has become the fastest growing of all bariatric procedures and continues at the highest rate today [3]. Outside of the six fundamental bariatric surgical procedures that have predominated the last fifty years, there is still ongoing research into improvements in the treatment of obesity and metabolic disorders. Endoluminal procedures are at the forefront of research and include devices to restrict and occupy space within the GI tract to decrease calorie absorption (balloons). Other methods include sleeves to recreate surgical gastric bypass and neural-hormonal limiting devices.

Review Questions

1. Metabolic surgery was fathered at the University of Minnesota in which decade?

   A. 1890s
   B. 1920s
   C. 1950s
   D. 2000s

2. There are six principal bariatric surgery procedures. Which is considered to pose the least risk of *severe* complications?

   A. Sleeve gastrectomy
   B. Roux-en-Y gastric bypass
   C. Adjustable gastric band
   D. Duodenal switch

3. All of the following are known complications of jejunoileal bypass except:

   A. Calcium oxalate kidney stones
   B. Vitamin D, calcium, and vitamin deficiencies
   C. Excessive weight loss
   D. Gas-bloat syndrome

Answers

1. The answer is *C*. The original bariatric surgeries were completed in the 1950s by Dr. Varco. The extent and types of surgical interventions for weight loss have developed since.
2. The answer is *C*. All surgeries carry a risk of complication, and metabolic surgeries are no exception. Adjustable gastric bands placed

laparoscopically pose the least risk of *severe* complication, but it is important to remember that multiple complications still exist and can even be prevalent. Patients with an AGB require the most strict follow-up as band adjustments are often necessary. Band slippage and erosion are the most common complications and both require urgent surgical correction. The most common complication of sleeve gastrectomy is staple line leak. Duodenal switch and gastric bypass both leave patients with anastomoses which can suffer from leaks, breakdown, or ulceration. Internal herniation becomes a possibility and can lead to disastrous complications.

3. The answer is *C*. Despite providing reliable excess weight loss and resolution of hyperlipidemia, the jejunoileal bypass also led to many early and late complications. Electrolyte imbalances, vitamin deficiencies, diarrhea, gas-bloat syndrome, oxalate kidney stones, fatty infiltration and degeneration of the liver, and even altered mentation were known in many patients. Loss of excess weight is an intended consequence of the JI bypass and not considered a complication.

References

1. Buchwald H (2014) The evolution of metabolic/bariatric surgery. Obes Surg 24:1126–1135
2. Flum DR et al (2009) Perioperative safety in the longitudinal assessment of bariatric surgery. N Engl J Med 361:445–454
3. Sunborn M (2014) Laparoscopic revolution in bariatric surgery. World J Gastroenterol 20:15135–15143

The Obesity Epidemic

4

Eve Bruneau

According the World Health Organization (WHO), obesity has doubled worldwide since 1980 and has become the leading cause of preventable deaths in the United States [1]. In 2013, the American Medical Association declared obesity a disease [2]. This epidemic has increased healthcare costs and put the population at risk for developing diabetes, cardiovascular disease, osteoarthritis, and some cancers [3, 4]. It's a difficult healthcare and social dilemma, with an obese and overweight population experiencing social stigmata, prejudice, and work discrimination [1, 3].

Obesity is an increasing global public health problem. A body mass index (BMI) greater than or equal to 25 is defined as overweight, greater than or equal to 30 is obese [3]. The WHO reports 13 % of the population being obese with 11 % of men and 15 % of women [1]. In 2013, 42 million children under the age of 5 were overweight or obese. Developing countries have a rise in low- and middle-income populations with obesity, and the rate of increase in childhood obesity is 30 % higher than that of developed countries. Obesity kills more people than underweight worldwide [1].

The increase in the overweight and obese population has not only taken a toll on world health, but contributes to rising healthcare costs, especially in the United States. In 1998 the medical costs were as high as $78.5 billion. More than half of this was funded by Medicare and Medicaid. Research has shown that there has been over a $40 billion increase in medical spending through 2006, with projections that these numbers could more than triple in the future [4].

Studies have shown that overweight individuals experience discrimination and stigmata, exacerbating poor eating habits and lower levels of physical exercise. There is an increasing biased attitude against obesity, contributing to reduced educational attainment, employment, and personal relationships [5]. These biased views extend into the healthcare field, where patients avoid follow-up appointments

E. Bruneau, DO
Department of General Surgery, Rowan University, Stratford, NJ, USA
e-mail: bruneaev@rowan.edu

© Springer International Publishing Switzerland 2017
A. Loveitt et al. (eds.), *Passing the Certified Bariatric Nurses Exam*,
DOI 10.1007/978-3-319-41703-5_4

and feel embarrassed to undress. Some members of the healthcare community perceive obese patients as lazy and lacking willpower and self-discipline [5]. It is important to eliminate these biases and discrimination and treat obesity as a disease to give the patient the best chances of weight loss and overall physical and mental health improvement.

The world is faced with a disease that is rampant and effects all ages, races, and socioeconomic classes. This disease takes a toll on the patient's physical, mental, and social health, as well as burdening the healthcare system with rising costs. Overweight and obese people need to be treated without bias, and the first step toward achieving a healthier life is weight loss. Weight-loss surgery, as detailed in this book, is an option to help address the global obesity dilemma.

Review Questions

1. The WHO states that developed countries have a higher rate of obesity in children than developing countries. True or False?

    A. True
    B. False

2. A 45-year-old female has a BMI of 28. What is her BMI classification?

    A. Normal weight
    B. Underweight
    C. Overweight
    D. Obese

3. When was obesity recognized as a disease in the United States?

    A. 1999
    B. 2013
    C. 2001
    D. 1975

Answers

1. The answer is *B*, false: Developing countries have a higher rate of obesity in children, at 30 % higher than developed.
2. The answer is *C*, overweight: A BMI of <18.5 is underweight, 18.5–24.9 is normal weight, 25–29.9 is overweight, and >30 is obese.
3. The answer is *B*, 2013. The American Medical Association recognized obesity as a disease in 2013.

References

1. World Health Organization. Obesity and overweight. 2015. [Online]. Available: http://www.who.int/mediacentre/factsheets/fs311/en/. Accessed 1 May 2016
2. Pollack A. The A.M.A. Recognizes obesity in a disease. The New York Times, 18 June 2013
3. Nguyen NT, Blackstone RP, Morton JM et al (2015) The ASMBS textbook of bariatric surgery. Springer, New York
4. Finkelstein EA et al (2009) Annual medical spending attributable to obesity: payer-and service-specific estimates. Health Aff (Millwood) 28(5):w822–w831
5. Budd GM (2011) Health care professionals' attitudes about obesity: an integrative review. Appl Nurs Res 23(3):127–137

Indications for Bariatric Surgery

5

Eve Bruneau

In order for a patient to be considered for weight-loss surgery, they must be evaluated by a multidisciplinary team. Surgical, medical, psychiatric, and nutritional experts perform thorough evaluations prior to surgery. Clearance from all these specialties optimizes results in weight loss, while providing the safest scenario for the patient perioperatively, postoperatively, and long term.

Body mass index (BMI) is used to measure body fat based on weight and height (Table 5.1). According to the NIH, potential candidates for bariatric surgery must have a BMI that exceeds 40 or BMIs between 35 and 40 with high-risk comorbidities and lifestyle limiting obesity-induced physical conditions (Tables 5.2 and 5.3). Traditionally age ranges have been 18–65 years old although some centers perform procedures in both pediatric and geriatric candidates [1].

Studies have shown that morbid obesity poses higher perioperative risks. The Obesity Surgery Mortality Risk Score (OS-MRS) predicts the 90-day mortality risk after gastric bypass surgery. It looks at five preoperative variables (Table 5.4). The OS-MRS aids in risk stratification when preoperatively assessing whether bariatric surgery is a safe option for weight loss [1].

In the past, patients with HIV were not considered candidates for weight-loss surgery; however, new antiviral therapies have increased life expectancy and decreased viral load. Some studies have shown safety and efficacy in well-controlled HIV patients [1].

As for patients with psychiatric disorders, bariatric surgery has been proven to be successful. Active psychosis should be treated, and a full psychiatric evaluation and clearance must be done preoperatively before any surgical intervention.

The bariatric population already possesses comorbidities such as hypertension, hyperlipidemia, obstructive sleep apnea, and diabetes, which place them in a higher perioperative risk category. Without proper multidisciplinary clearance, these

E. Bruneau, DO
Department of General Surgery, Rowan University, Stratford, NJ, USA
e-mail: bruneaev@rowan.edu

© Springer International Publishing Switzerland 2017
A. Loveitt et al. (eds.), *Passing the Certified Bariatric Nurses Exam*,
DOI 10.1007/978-3-319-41703-5_5

Table 5.1 Body mass index categories

BMI categories	BMI
Underweight	<18.5
Normal weight	18.5–24.9
Overweight	25–29.9
Obese	>30

Table 5.2 Absolute and relative contraindications to bariatric surgery [1, 2]

Absolute	Relative
Contraindications to general anesthesia	Uncontrolled drug or alcohol dependence
Uncorrectable coagulopathy	Cirrhosis with portal hypertension
Pregnancy	End-stage lung disease
	Active cancer
	Unstable coronary artery disease
	Heart failure

Table 5.3 Comorbidities associated with morbid obesity [2]

Hypertension	Nephrotic syndrome
Coronary artery disease	Thrombophlebitis
Heart failure	Wound infections or dehiscence
Venous stasis ulcers	Sexual hormone dysfunction
Diabetes and insulin intolerance	Necrotizing subcutaneous infections
Degenerative osteoarthritis	Stress urinary incontinence
Cholelithiasis	Gastroesophageal reflux disease
Polycystic ovarian syndrome (PCOS)	Respiratory insufficiency of obesity (Pickwickian syndrome)
Pseudotumor cerebri	Obesity hypoventilation syndrome
Increased intra-abdominal pressure	Obesity sleep apnea syndrome
Nonalcoholic steatohepatitis	Venous disease
Pulmonary embolism	

patients are not only at risk of suffering failed weight loss but are also put at risk of morbidities such as myocardial infarction, stroke, psychological breakdown, and even mortality. Multidisciplinary evaluation prior to weight-loss surgery creates the safest and most optimal environment for a patient to achieve and maintain their weight-loss goal.

Table 5.4   The obesity surgery mortality risk score

Body mass index >50 kg/m^2
Male gender
Hypertension

Increased risk of pulmonary embolism:
    Previous thrombus
    Previous pulmonary embolism
    Inferior vena cava filter
    Right heart failure
    Obesity hypoventilation syndrome

Age >/= 45 years

Score	Mortality risk (%)
0–1	0.2
2–3	1.1
4–5	2.4

Each variable equals 1 point, resulting in a score of 0–5 [3]

Review Questions

1. A 45-year-old female presents to her family physician for her yearly physical. Her BMI is 36 and has been steadily rising over the past few years. She inquires about weight-loss surgery. What should her physician advise?

   A. Refer her to a bariatric surgeon.
   B. Tell her that her BMI is high and needs to attempt weight loss through diet modification and exercise.
   C. Advise the patient that her BMI is within normal range and will continue to monitor on her next annual exam.
   D. Prescribe a weight-loss medication.

2. All of the following are considered comorbidities associated with morbid obesity EXCEPT:

   A. Diabetes
   B. Hypertension
   C. Pseudotumor cerebri
   D. Asthma

3. A 47-year-old male with a BMI of 62 has struggled with his weight for years. He has failed to lose weight, despite diet modification and exercise. He has a history of hypertension controlled with medication,

diabetes, osteoarthritis, and alcohol abuse. Which of the following is a relative contraindication to him undergoing bariatric surgery.

A. BMI of 42
B. Alcohol abuse
C. Male sex
D. Hypertension

4. A 65-year-old woman with a medical history of deep vein thrombus and hypertension and a BMI of 43 is being evaluated for bariatric surgery. She asks her physician what her mortality risk is. According to the OS-MRS, what is her risk of mortality?

A. 0%
B. 0.2%
C. 1.1%
D. 10%

Answers

1. The answer is *B*. Patients should attempt weight loss through lifestyle and diet modifications before exploring bariatric surgery. If that fails, then they can be evaluated by a multidisciplinary team to determine whether or not they are a candidate for weight-loss surgery.
2. The answer is *D*. Asthma is not considered a comorbidity associated with obesity. Please refer to Table 5.3 for the list of comorbidities.
3. The answer is *B*. Alcohol and drug dependence are relative contraindications to bariatric surgery. Refer to Table 5.2 for the complete list.
4. The answer is *C*. Her risk of mortality is 1.1% given her age, history of thrombus, and hypertension. Her calculated variable score is 3, placing her at 1.1% perioperative risk of mortality. Refer to Table 5.4.

References

1. Nguyen NT, Blackstone RP, Morton JM et al (2015) The ASMBS textbook of bariatric surgery. Springer, New York
2. Mullholand MW, et al Greenfield's: surgery and scientific principles & practice, 5th edn. LWW; Philadelphia, 2012
3. Vogler GP et al (1995) Influences of genes and shared family environment on adult body mass index assessed in an adoption study by a comprehensive path model. Int J Obes Relat Metab Disord 19:40–45

Basic Anatomy and Physiology of the Gastrointestinal Tract

6

Eve Bruneau

The gastrointestinal tract begins at the mouth and ends at the anus (Fig. 6.1). Its purpose is to mechanically and enzymatically digest food, absorb nutrients and water, protect the body from microbial invasion, and expel feces. Food enters the mouth where mechanical and enzymatic digestion begins and then is propelled down the esophagus and into the stomach where digestion continues. As the food bolus passes through the small intestine, further digestion and absorption take place with the help of enzymes secreted by the stomach, small intestine, liver, and pancreas. The majority of water absorption and formation of feces occur in the large intestine, until it is temporarily stored in the rectum and defecated through the anus [1].

6.1 Esophagus

The esophagus is divided into three regions: cervical (C6 to T1), thoracic (T1 to the esophageal hiatus of the diaphragm), and abdominal (esophageal hiatus to the cardia of the stomach). It passes slightly right to the aorta and goes through the diaphragm slightly left [2].

Blood Supply

Cervical: branches of the inferior thyroid artery and vein.
Thoracic: branches directly off the aorta and the accessory hemiazygos or left bra- chiocephalic vein.
Abdominal: branches of the left gastric artery and vein.

E. Bruneau, DO
Department of General Surgery, Rowan University, Stratford, NJ, USA
e-mail: bruneaev@rowan.edu

© Springer International Publishing Switzerland 2017
A. Loveitt et al. (eds.), *Passing the Certified Bariatric Nurses Exam*,
DOI 10.1007/978-3-319-41703-5_6

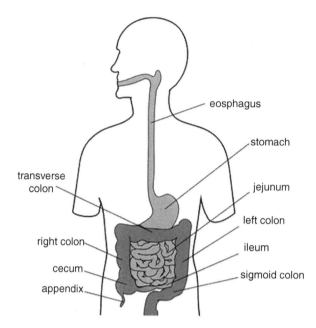

Fig. 6.1 Basic anatomy of the GI tract

Nerves Left and right vagus nerve, left running anterior, and right running posterior.

6.2   Stomach

The stomach is divided into the fundus, cardia, body, pylorus, and antrum (Fig. 6.2). The stomach is responsible for mechanical and enzymatic digestion of food. Numerous hormones are secreted (Table 6.1).

Blood Supply

Arteries: blood supply originates from the celiac artery. Branches include left and right gastric, left and right gastroepiploic, short gastric, and gastroduodenal arteries [3].

Veins: the corresponding veins drain into the portal or superior mesenteric venous systems [1].

Nerves Parasympathetic supply: left vagus nerve runs anteriorly, right vagus nerve runs posteriorly. The sympathetic supply consists of spinal segments T5–T10 [2].

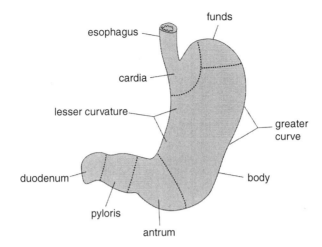

Fig. 6.2 Stomach anatomy

Table 6.1 Hormones of the GI tract

Hormone	Source	Stimuli for release	Major activities
Somatostatin	Antrum, duodenum, pancreatic islet cells	Acid in the stomach	Acts on parietal cells in the stomach to reduce acid secretion and prevents secretion of gastrin, secretin, and histamine
Gastrin	G cells (antrum)	Amino acids, acetylcholine	Stimulates gastric acid secretion and proliferation of gastric epithelium
CCK	Duodenum	Fatty acids, amino acids in the small intestine	Stimulates release of pancreatic enzymes and gallbladder contraction
Secretin	Duodenum	Acid in the duodenum	Stimulates secretion of water and bicarbonate from the pancreas and bile ducts
Ghrelin	Stomach, duodenum, jejunum	Empty stomach	Stimulates appetite/feeding
Motilin	Duodenum, jejunum	Fasting state	Motility of stomach and small intestine
Gastric inhibitory polypeptide	K cells in the duodenum and jejunum	Fat and glucose in the small intestine	Inhibits gastric secretion and motility and increases insulin release

6.3   Small Intestine

The small intestine is divided into the duodenum, jejunum, and ileum. Enzymes excreted from the pancreas and liver mix with the chyme propelled out the stomach and continue to digest the food. This is where absorption of essential nutrients begins. Hormones associated with the small bowel are listed in Table 6.1.

6.3.1   Duodenum

The duodenum has the first (bulb), second (descending), third (transverse), and fourth (ascending) portions. The pancreas drains into the duodenum through the accessory and major pancreatic ducts at the major and minor papilla located in the descending portion. The small intestine is the site of fat-soluble vitamin absorption (vitamins A, D, E, and K).

Blood Supply

Arteries: the gastroduodenal and superior pancreaticoduodenal branches off the hepatic and inferior pancreaticoduodenal branch off the superior mesenteric
Veins: superior mesenteric vein

Nerves Derived from the celiac plexus [1].

6.3.2   Jejunum

The jejunum contains villi to maximize water and nutrient absorption.

Blood Supply

Arteries: jejunal arteries are branches of the superior mesenteric artery and have long vasa recta.
Veins: the veins run with the corresponding arteries, draining into the superior mesenteric artery.

Nerves Sympathetic fibers form Auerbach's and Meissner's plexuses [1].

6.3.3   Ileum

Like the jejunum, the ileum contains villi and is responsible for absorption of B12 and folate (terminal ileum) and bile acids [2].

Blood Supply

Arteries: ileal arteries are branches of the superior mesenteric artery with short vasa recta.

Veins: the veins run with the corresponding arteries, draining into the superior mesenteric artery.

Nerves Sympathetic fibers form Auerbach's and Meissner's plexuses [1, 2]

6.4   Colon and Rectum

The colon is comprised of the haustra, taeniae coli, and appendices epiploicae. The taeniae coli are in between the haustra, which are pockets of the colon wall. The appendices epiploicae are the fat appendages on the colonic serosa. The colon wall consists of five layers: mucosa, submucosa, circular and longitudinal muscle layers, and serosa. The colon has columnar epithelium, with crypts and goblet cells, and unlike the small bowel, there are no villi. The rectum does not have haustra or epiploicae, and the beginning of the rectum is where the taeniae coli converge [1, 2].

The colon is responsible for water, sodium, and chloride absorption, secreting potassium and bicarbonate. Liquid stool becomes formed feces, and it is moved through the colon. Colonic flora, such as *B. fragilis* and *E coli*, aid in the absorption and digestion of molecules, immunity, and protection against noncommensal bacteria. Colonic bacteria also produce vitamin B12 and K [2].

The rectum is the final portion of the large intestine, beginning at the rectosigmoid junction at the level of the sacral promontory. It acts as temporary storage of stool before it is defecated through the anal canal. Feces are expelled through the rectum by peristaltic waves, passing through the internal and external sphincter and out the anus [1, 2].

Blood Supply

Arteries:
   Cecum: ileocecal artery
   Appendix: appendiceal from the ileocecal artery
   Right colon: right colic artery
   Transverse colon: middle colic
   Left colon: left colic
   Sigmoid: sigmoid artery
   Rectum: superior and inferior rectal arteries
Veins: the veins run with the corresponding arteries, draining into the superior and inferior mesenteric arteries [1, 3].

Nerves Right colon: parasympathetic innervation arises from the right vagus nerve. Sympathetic innervation from lower thoracic segments in the thoracic splanchnic nerves, celiac, and superior mesenteric plexuses.

Left colon and rectum: parasympathetic innervation arises from the S1 to S4 spinal cord segments. Sympathetic innervation from L1 to L3 spinal segments [1, 2].

Review Questions

1. All of the following are branches of the superior mesenteric artery except:

    A. Left colic
    B. Appendiceal artery
    C. Right colic
    D. Ileocecal artery

2. All of the following vitamins are fat soluble except:

    A. Vitamin A
    B. Vitamin K
    C. Vitamin C
    D. Vitamin D

3. What is the anatomical landmark associated with rectosigmoid junction?

    A. Sacral promontory
    B. Iliac crest
    C. Thoracolumbar junction
    D. Origin of the inferior mesenteric artery

4. These are all hormones secreted by the duodenum except:

    A. Secretin
    B. Gastrin
    C. Somatostatin
    D. Motilin

5. An 85-year-old female suffered an infarct to her small bowel, resulting in resection of over 60 cm of the ileum. What is she at risk of developing?

    A. Dehydration
    B. Vitamin B12 deficiency
    C. Diarrhea
    D. Vitamin C deficiency

Answers

1. The answer is *A*, left colic. The branches of the superior mesenteric artery are the ileocolic, right and middle colic, and ileal and jejunal arteries. The branches of the inferior mesenteric artery are the left colic and sigmoid artery and superior rectal artery.

2. The answer is *C*, vitamin C. Fat-soluble vitamins include vitamins A, D, E, and K (2).
3. The answer is *A*, sacral promontory. The rectosigmoid junction is located at the sacral promontory where the taeniae coli converge.
4. The answer is *B*, gastrin. The stomach secretes gastrin in response to the presence of acetylcholine and amino acids. The duodenum secretes cholecystokinin, secretin, ghrelin, motilin, somatostatin, and gastric inhibitory polypeptide.
5. The answer is *B*, vitamin B12 deficiency. The majority of water resorption is in the colon. Diarrhea is not associated with a shortened ileum, but Vitamin B12 is mainly absorbed in the ileum.

References

1. Susan Standring. Gray's anatomy, 41st edn. Elsevier: London, UK; 2016
2. Mullholand MW, et al. Greenfield's: surgery and scientific principles & practice, 5th edn. LWWL: London, UK; 2012
3. Gilroy AM, et al. Atlas of anatomy 1st edn., Thieme Medical Publisher, Inc., New York; 2008

Medical Strategies for Weight Loss

7

Andrew Loveitt

Most patients who turn to weight-loss surgery have struggled with their weight throughout their adolescent and adult lives. Initial attempts at weight loss include dietary modifications and exercise. While these may lead to some success in the short term, long-term success is despairingly rare. The bariatric nurse must be familiar with these concepts and their outcomes to adequately council the bariatric patient as well as understand what they have been through.

The essential principle of weight loss, energy out > energy in, is easy for the patient to understand. However, it is essential to recognize that there are a multitude of other factors at play. Energy balance is centrally regulated by the hypothalamus and brainstem using both hormonal and neural pathways which in turn are affected by a complex balance of genetic, social, behavioral, and physiologic signals [1].

7.1 Energy Intake

Mechanical signals, including stretching of the esophagus and stomach during meals, act directly on the brainstem and hypothalamus.

Leptin is a hormone released by fat cells signaling the amount of energy stored in the body. It acts to suppress appetite and increase energy expenditure. Obese individuals have been shown to be resistant to this hormone making it a potential target for weight-loss therapies [1].

Ghrelin is a hormone released by the stomach which has been shown to stimulate food intake in animal and human studies. It has been labeled a "hunger hormone." Levels increase during fasting and decrease after eating. While the overall level of

A. Loveitt, DO
Department of General Surgery, Rowan University, Stratford, NJ, USA
e-mail: Loveitan@rowan.edu

© Springer International Publishing Switzerland 2017
A. Loveitt et al. (eds.), *Passing the Certified Bariatric Nurses Exam*,
DOI 10.1007/978-3-319-41703-5_7

ghrelin in obese individuals is reduced, they do not experience the same postprandial drop in levels [1].

Other hormones implicated in the hunger-satiation response include cholecystokinin, peptide YY, and glucagon-like peptide-1. While research continues, to date,
there have been no effective therapies developed which take advantage of our
increasing understanding in this area.

7.2 Energy Expenditure

The body requires a baseline amount of energy to undergo its basic metabolic
actions, this is known as basal metabolic rate (BMR). The body will require additional energy for any physical activity beyond the BMR. When counseling a patient
on weight loss, it is important to determine what their daily energy expenditure is so
that they can tailor their intake. There are numerous equations available; however,
the Mifflin-St. Jeor is easy to calculate [2]:

$$BMR = \left[Constant + (9.99 \times Weight) + (6.25 \times Height) - (4.92 \times Age) \right]$$
$$\text{The constant being 5 for males and } -161 \text{ for females}$$

The BMR is then multiplied by an activity factor to arrive at total energy expenditure: 1.2, sedentary; 1.375, mild activity; 1.55, moderate activity; 1.7, heavy activity; 1.9, extreme activity.

For office purposes it may be more efficient to arrive at a reasonable estimate by
first determining the ideal body weight (IBW) based on height:

IBW Male = 106 lbs for first 5 feet + 6 lbs for each additional inch in height

IBW Female = 100 lbs for first 5 feet + 5 lbs for each additional inch in height

Once IBW is determined, it can be multiplied by 12–13 for women and 13–15 for
men to arrive at a reasonable goal for daily caloric intake [3].

7.3 Assessing Weight Loss

Once a patient begins on their weight-loss journey (whether it be through medical
or surgical intervention), it is imperative to track their progress. Journals are highly
recommended to track patient's activity and dietary habits as well as their progress.
While overall weight loss is an important metric, percent of excess weight loss
(%EWL) is more pertinent and can be calculated as:

$$\%EWL = \left((\text{preintervention weight} - \text{current weight}) \div (\text{preintervention weight} - IBW) \right)$$

7.4   Nonsurgical Interventions for Weight Loss

Successful weight loss must start with a multimodal approach including diet, exercise, and behavioral modification. A full history and physical should include [1]:

1. History of weight gain and loss
2. Medications which contribute to weight gain (steroids, antipsychotic agents)
3. Previous attempts at weight loss
4. Patterns of food intake
5. Physical activity levels

7.4.1   Diet

Patients with a BMI <35 should seek to reduce their caloric intake by 500 kcal/day. This will generally result in loss of 1 pound per week and a 10 % weight reduction in 6 months. If the BMI is >35, a reduction of 500–1000 kcal/day should be sought to achieve weight loss of 1–2 pounds per week. Currently a low-carbohydrate, high-protein diet is recommended as protein is thought to increase satiety [1]. Other recommendations to increase satiation include encouragement of five small meals per day and chewing food 20–30 times per bite. Protein supplements can be used as meal replacements.

7.4.2   Exercise

A high volume and physical intensity level of exercise is required to induce weight loss; however, it should be encouraged in all patients who are physically able and plays a large role in long-term weight management. A journal should be established to track the patient's progress. An exercise "prescription" can be given to the patient based on the FITT (frequency, intensity, time, and type) principle. Special considerations must be taken when prescribing exercise programs to obese and should take into account their cardiovascular, pulmonary, and musculoskeletal status. Adjuncts such as aquatic exercise programs have proven successful in reducing musculoskeletal complications which can limit an obese patient's ability to comply with an exercise program [4]. Sixty to ninety minutes per day of moderate-to-vigorous intensity physical activity is suggested to maintain weight loss [1].

7.4.3   Behavioral Therapy

Personal, psychological, and social cues contribute greatly to our eating habits and often impede long-term weight-loss success. Strategies of behavior control include avoiding stimuli that lead to eating, activity, and consumption logs to help identify these cues and social support. Group therapy has proven successful and should be continued long term [1].

7.4.4 Pharmacological Therapy

Indications for consideration of pharmacological therapy for weight loss include BMI >30 and BMI >27 with the presence of an obesity-related complication including type 2 diabetes, hypertension, and dyslipidemia [1]. Many medications have been withdrawn because of side effects. Currently approved drugs include [3]:

- Orlistat – inhibits gastric and pancreatic lipases limiting the digestion and absorption of fat. It is recommended for use for up to 6 months along with a weight-loss program. There is an over-the-counter formulation sold as Alli. Side effects include fatty/oily stool, fecal urgency and incontinence, flatulence, and decreased absorption of fat-soluble vitamins.
- Lorcaserin (Belviq) – a moderately selective serotonin 2C receptor blocker. It acts directly on the brain to decrease appetite. Trials show a 3 % increase in weight loss over placebo. Side effects include headache, dizziness, fatigue, and GI complaints.
- Phentermine-topiramate (Qsymia) – mechanism of action is not known. Clinical studies have shown a 9 % weight loss over placebo. Serious side effects have been established including birth defects (cleft lip and palate), tachycardia, suicidal ideation, and other neurological effects.

Despite intensive medical and pharmacological therapy, few people are able to successfully maintain weight loss. While many will eventually turn to bariatric surgery, there are multiple reasons to first attempt medical weight loss; it is low risk, is often needed for insurance authorization, and can enhance the safety of the surgical procedure by lowering cardiopulmonary risk factors as well as reducing the size of the liver to create a technically less challenging procedure.

Review Questions
1. A 46-year-old female who is 5′2″ and weighs 300 lbs presents to your clinic. She has had multiple unsuccessful weight-loss attempts in the past. She is interested in a medically directed weight-loss attempt. What is her ideal body weight?

   A. 95 lbs
   B. 105 lbs
   C. 110 lbs
   D. 115 lbs

2. What is the suggested daily caloric intake to achieve weight loss in the above patient?

   A. 1000 kcal/day.
   B. 1320–1430 kcal/day.
   C. 500–1000 kcal less than previous intake.
   D. All patients should be on a 2000 kcal/day diet.
   E. B and C are correct.

3. The patient's initial attempts at weight loss fail, and she is started on a medication as an adjunct. She returns to the clinic complaining she is now having fatty, foul-smelling stools. What is your recommendation?

   A. This is a common side effect of Orlistat, and she should continue on the medication if the side effects are tolerable.
   B. She should be sent to see a gastroenterologist; this is likely the onset of celiac disease.
   C. Her stool should be tested for C. diff.
   D. Her Qsymia should be stopped.

4. Despite the addition of Orlistat, the patient still does not achieve her desired weight loss and she elects to undergo a laparoscopic sleeve gastrectomy. At her 6-month follow-up, she is down to a weight of 210 pounds. What is her percent of excess weight loss?

   A. 30 %
   B. 38 %
   C. 42 %
   D. 47 %

5. Ghrelin has been described as the "hunger hormone." What levels would you expect to find in an obese patient while fasting? After eating?

   A. Increased with fasting, unchanged after eating
   B. Increased with fasting, decreased after eating
   C. Reduced with fasting, increased after eating
   D. Reduced with fasting, unchanged after eating
   E. Reduced with fasting, reduced after eating

Answers

1. The answer is C. Ideal body weight for a female is calculated as 100 lbs for the first 5 ft in height plus an additional 5 pounds for each additional inch. The patient is 5 ft (100 lbs) +2 in. (5×2 = 10 lbs) which results in an ideal body weight of 110 lbs.

2. The answer is E. The patient's ideal body weight of 110 lbs can be multiplied by 12–13 for an easy estimate of recommended caloric intake per day. Alternatively, simply asking the patient to withhold 500–1000 kcal/

day from their previous diet will be an effective first step and should lead to 1–2 lbs of weight loss per week.

3. The answer is *A*. Orlistat is known to cause fatty, foul-smelling stools as it limits the absorption of fat in the GI system. Since the drug itself is not absorbed, there are limited systemic effects. If the patient can tolerate her change in bowel habits, she may continue the drug. While celiac disease and C. diff could cause these findings, they are less likely given the clinical scenario. Qsymia's side effect profile includes birth defects and neurological effects, not GI symptoms.

4. The answer is *D*. %EWL for this patient is calculated using 300 pounds as the preintervention weight, 210 pounds as the current weight, and 110 pounds as the ideal body weight:

$$(300-210) \div (300-110) = 47\ \%$$

5. The answer is *D*. In obese individuals the ghrelin level is low at baseline; however, it does not drop significantly even after eating as it would in an individual of appropriate weight.

References

1. Cowley M, Brown W, Considine R (2016) Obesity. In: Endocrinology: adult and pediatric. Elsevier Saunders, Philadelphia, pp 468–478
2. Mifflin MD, St Jeor ST, Hill LA et al (1990) A new predictive equation for resting energy expenditure in healthy individuals. Am J Clin Nutr 51(2):241–247
3. Rakel R, Rakel D (2016) Obesity. In: Textbook of family medicine. Elsevier Saunders, Philadelphia, pp 867–890
4. Boidin M, Lapierre G, Tanir LP et al (2015) Effect of aquatic interval training with Mediterranean diet counseling in obese patients: results of a preliminary study. Ann Phys Rehabil Med 58(5):269–275

Restrictive Versus Malabsorptive Procedures in Bariatric Surgery

8

William Stembridge

Throughout the evolution of bariatric and metabolic surgery, two primary mechanisms have been identified as generating the loss of excess body weight. While the specific surgical manipulations of the gastrointestinal tract and surgeons performing them are many and varied, the two underlying principles at work are *restriction* of ingested food and *malabsorption* of ingested food. Modern metabolic and bariatric operations all employ one or both of these principles.

Restrictive surgeries entail physically limiting the quantity of food a patient is able to ingest. This is typically accomplished by limiting the size and capacity of the stomach while leaving the remainder of the gastrointestinal tract intact. The two most common procedures performed today of a restrictive nature are the sleeve gastrectomy and adjustable gastric band. While the majority of the stomach is surgically and permanently excised during a laparoscopic sleeve gastrectomy, the organ is partially constricted using an inflatable band during a laparoscopic adjustable gastric band application. Following either surgery, patients reach a feeling of satiety much sooner while eating and consume a substantially smaller portion of food. With sleeve gastrectomy procedures, hormonal changes occur as well due to excision of the aspect of the stomach responsible for the production of several systemic hormones [1]. This will be discussed in a later chapter.

Malabsorption of calories and nutrients occurs when a portion of the gastrointestinal tract is bypassed or removed. The gut is exposed to ingested foods for a shorter distance, and therefore less calories and nutrients are able to be absorbed. Typically, there is also a diversion of digestive enzymes from the liver, pancreas, and gallbladder such that they meet with ingested food at a later portion of the GI tract and further decrease the digestion and availability of food and nutrients for absorption. There are no purely malabsorptive bariatric surgeries being performed in modern

W. Stembridge, DO
Department of General Surgery, Rowan University, Stratford, NJ, USA
e-mail: stembrwi@rowan.edu

© Springer International Publishing Switzerland 2017
A. Loveitt et al. (eds.), *Passing the Certified Bariatric Nurses Exam*,
DOI 10.1007/978-3-319-41703-5_8

33

practice. The duodeno-ileal bypass was performed from the 1950s to 1970s and represented a purely malabsorptive surgery but was fraught with complication [1]. Roux-en-Y gastric bypass and biliopancreatic diversion with duodenal switch are two contemporary surgeries that are considered to be malabsorptive in nature but also have restrictive aspects. After the stomach is divided in either operation, the ileum is also separated and anastomosed such that ingested food and digestive enzymes remain on separate tracks until a final, shortened common channel where digestion and absorption of nutrients can occur. These efforts to cause both restriction and malabsorption typically yield a higher percentage of excess weight loss but also can lead to additional and separate complications. Patients having a gastric bypass or duodenal switch must be advised to supplement their diets with vitamins and nutrients to avoid deficiency [2].

Review Questions

1. A patient presents for evaluation prior to undergoing bariatric surgery. Her BMI is 52 and she suffers from non-insulin-dependent diabetes mellitus, hypertension, and obstructive sleep apnea. Which of the following operations would she *least* likely be offered?

   A. Adjustable gastric band
   B. Sleeve gastrectomy
   C. Roux-en-Y gastric bypass
   D. Biliopancreatic diversion with duodenal switch

2. What is the mechanism of weight loss in a Roux-en-Y gastric bypass?

   A. Restrictive
   B. Malabsorptive
   C. Both
   D. None of the above

3. Which of the procedures below are *least* likely to result in nutritional deficiencies?

   A. Roux-en-Y gastric bypass
   B. Adjustable gastric band
   C. Sleeve gastrectomy
   D. Biliopancreatic diversion with duodenal switch

4. What is the mechanism that leads to weight loss after the sleeve gastrectomy?

   A. Restrictive
   B. Hormonal
   C. Malabsorptive
   D. A and B

1. The answer is *A*. While none of the above choices are technically wrong, patients with super morbid obesity and multiple comorbidities have been found to lose a greater percentage of excess body mass and have better resolution of the comorbidities when they undergo an operation which has a malabsorptive effect. This is especially true for diabetic patients. Therefore, the biliopancreatic diversion and Roux-en-Y gastric bypass would be preferable. A sleeve gastrectomy would lead to substantial weight loss and improvements in comorbidities but to a lesser extent. An adjustable gastric band requires very close follow-up and does the least to remedy comorbidities such as DM.

2. The answer is *C*. Roux-en-Y gastric bypass includes components of both restrictive and malabsorptive mechanisms of weight loss. The stomach is reduced to a small pouch, and biliopancreatic digestive enzymes are diverted from ingested food for the majority of the length of the small bowel.

3. The answer is *B*. The adjustable gastric band is a completely restrictive procedure and therefore is least likely to result in nutritional deficiencies as long as the patient eats a well-rounded diet. The sleeve gastrectomy has a low likelihood as well, but not as low as the band. The Roux-en-Y and biliopancreatic diversion both have malabsorptive components, and patients should be monitored closely for deficiencies.

4. The answer is *D*. The sleeve gastrectomy has been found to have significant hormonal effects which lead to almost immediate improvement in comorbidities such as hypertension and diabetes. The hormone effect also significantly improves satiety. There is also a restrictive component as the stomach is essentially being made into a narrow tube. There is no significant malabsorptive component.

References

1. Townsend CM, Sabiston DC (2004) Sabiston textbook of surgery: the biological basis of modern surgical practice. Saunders, Philadelphia
2. Valera-Mora M et al (2005) Predictors of weight loss and reversal of comorbidities in malabsorptive bariatric surgery. Am J Clin Nutr 81(6):1292–1297

Preoperative Evaluation of the Bariatric Surgery Patient

9

William Stembridge

As with any operative undertaking, a careful analysis of the risks and benefits of the planned bariatric surgical procedure must be made. The initial encounter between the patient and bariatric surgeon typically occurs as a result of referral, whether from another physician involved in the patient's care, a satisfied past patient, or research and self-referral. From this time, a careful bond is formed between the surgeon and patient to facilitate the safest and most efficient realization of the patient's weight loss goals. By its nature, bariatric surgery is performed only on an elective basis; as such a thorough preoperative evaluation is necessary to minimize the risk of undue complications. The goal of this evaluation and workup is not necessarily to uncover any and all underlying medical diseases but to identify, analyze, and account for any comorbidities which could affect the patient in the perioperative (surgery and 48 h after) and postoperative (30 days) periods. Well-proven indicators for increased risk of peri- and postoperative complication include American Society of Anesthesiologist classification, American Heart Association/American College of Cardiologist guidelines, age, and multiple other indications of underlying medical diseases such as diabetes mellitus, cardiovascular disease, and renal impairment. When deciding the extent of necessary preoperative workup, the patient's history and physical exam, the intended procedure, anesthesia plan (all laparoscopic bariatric surgeries are performed under general anesthesia), and the expected postoperative disposition are analyzed [1].

When a thorough history and physical exam reveal signs of underlying comorbid disease, which are increasingly common in the morbidly obese patient population, further workup is warranted. In the setting of uncontrolled or poorly controlled medical diseases, consultation to a medical internist and/or medical subspecialist can be exceedingly helpful. Common comorbid diseases and a general understanding of their workup and management will be discussed by organ system.

W. Stembridge, DO
Department of General Surgery, Rowan University, Stratford, NJ, USA
e-mail: stembrwi@rowan.edu

© Springer International Publishing Switzerland 2017
A. Loveitt et al. (eds.), *Passing the Certified Bariatric Nurses Exam*,
DOI 10.1007/978-3-319-41703-5_9

9.1   Cardiovascular

Approximately 30 % of patients undergoing surgery in the United States have significant coronary artery disease or a severe cardiac comorbidity. One in eight of
these will suffer a perioperative complication [2]. If a patient has a known history of
cardiac disease, he or she should receive a full evaluation and workup by his/her
existing cardiologist. Evaluation of the patient's functional status, presence of
symptoms, and the use of one of many accepted cardiac risk assessment guidelines
should be performed. Essential hypertension, pulmonary hypertension, left ventric-
ular hypertrophy, congestive heart failure, and ischemic heart disease are all found
at a higher frequency in morbidly obese patients. Patients with any of these factors
are eligible for beta-blocker therapy, and patients with two or more should undergo
further noninvasive cardiovascular testing prior to any elective operation [2]. Tests
that may be ordered include exercise or chemical stress test, echocardiogram, or
even direct coronary angiography in patients with a substantial cardiac history or
previous revascularization (catheterization with balloon angioplasty or bypass
graft). If warranted, elective bariatric surgery may be postponed in favor of having
coronary revascularization. In the setting of a recent myocardial infarction and subsequent revascularization, the risks of surgery and anesthesia are substantially elevated in the first six weeks, and elective operations are contraindicated during that
time. Patients with a history of coronary stenting require antiplatelet therapy and
will often be continued on aspirin and other medications such as clopidogrel or
ticagrelor [2].

9.2   Pulmonary

Obesity, obstructive sleep apnea (OSA), and obesity hypoventilation syndrome
(OHVS) are all substantial risks for perioperative complication. Most morbidly
obese patients suffer from OSA and OHVS. Many already follow with pulmonolo-
gists and are being treated. While weight reduction offers the greatest likelihood of
curing these diseases, the patients should still remain under the care of their pulmonary specialists during the pre-, peri-, and postoperative periods [3]. Careful history
taking and examination of patients who may not carry these diagnoses are critical as
they may have OSA and OHVS but not be diagnosed or properly treated. These
patients should also be sent to a pulmonologist for consultation and sleep study
evaluation. Treatments such as continuous positive pressure ventilation and bron-
chodilators will likely need to be continued before and after the surgery.

9.3   Renal

Evaluation for signs of renal dysfunction is of utmost importance in the patient
undergoing bariatric surgery. Patients with known renal impairment should be followed by their primary nephrologists. Occasionally, patients on renal replacement

therapy will undergo bariatric surgery and will therefore need hemodialysis treatments and close monitoring of their serum chemistry while in the hospital. Kidney disease raises the risks for cardiac events in the perioperative setting as well as many other complications [2]. Patients with renal disease will need electrocardiogram monitoring, and signs of heart failure or volume overload should be monitored. Dialysis and other medical interventions for electrolyte abnormalities such as hyperkalemia, hyperphosphatemia, hypocalcemia, and others may need to occur. Anemia of chronic kidney disease is also commonly present in such patients. The pharmacodynamics of many medication classes including opiate pain medications is typically prolonged in patients with renal impairment.

Even in the patient without existing renal impairment, preventing any insult to the kidneys is a concern in the bariatric patient. In the post- and perioperative periods, maintaining adequate intravascular volume can be challenging. Obese postoperative patients who have a difficult time taking adequate liquids by mouth pose a unique risk for hypovolemia and may require substantial intravenous fluid administrations. Further, nephrotoxic medications such as NSAIDs and several diuretic antihypertensive medications should generally be avoided. To avoid the need for invasive monitoring of volume status, strict vital signs and intake/output measurements are very important and will be closely followed by the bariatric surgeon.

9.4   Endocrine

A number of endocrine diseases and deficiencies play a role in the perioperative care of bariatric patients: most commonly diabetes mellitus, thyroid disorders, and adrenal disorders. With an increasing incidence in the general population, especially in the obese, as well as representing an indication for bariatric surgery, diabetes mellitus is a common and potentially complicated illness in the bariatric population. Patients should be carefully screened in the preoperative evaluation for signs and symptoms of DM to include neuropathy and retinopathy plus laboratory testing for signs of complications of DM such as nephropathy, cardiac disease, and peripheral vascular disease [3]. Adequate control of blood sugars, typically with the assistance of an internist or endocrinologist, is paramount. A serum hemoglobin A1c value can be drawn to assess the adequacy of blood sugar control over recent weeks. The patient will continue on his/her prescribed glucose control regimen in the preoperative period, which often requires subcutaneous injections of insulin. This regimen will be seen to change in the perioperative period as insulin resistance in type 2 diabetics begins to resolve almost immediately after bariatric surgery. Most patients will be able to omit oral antihyperglycemic medications by the time of discharge and will see substantial reductions in their insulin needs as well. Typically, surgeons will instruct patients to use one half to one third of their regularly prescribed insulin doses the evening and morning of surgery to account for prolonged NPO status. Oral medications are held the day of surgery and often discontinued. The medication metformin should be noted to increase the risk of acute kidney injury, especially in the setting of hypovolemia or IV contrast administration. While in the hospital, frequent finger stick blood glucose values (every six hours) with an insulin sliding scale are prudent for following glucose values in the perioperative period. Any circumstances of overt hypoglycemia should beckon a call to the physician and prompt treatment with oral supplementation (juice, glucose) or intravenous dextrose for a symptomatic patient.

Thyroid hormone replacement therapy is typically continued and not altered in the perioperative time frame. A thyroid-stimulating hormone value and likely further serum thyroid studies may be ordered to insure tight control. Patients requiring chronic medications, especially corticosteroids, for adrenal insufficiency will need special stress-dose steroids to tolerate the operation and will likely need to receive medications while in the hospital. Close follow-up with an internist or endocrinologist both before and after bariatric surgery is helpful as the conditions above should be medically managed as tightly as possible before the operation and will have further changes in dosing postoperatively, especially in regard to DM medications.

9.5   Hepatobiliary

Patients in whom a clinical suspicion exists for underlying hepatic impairment should be investigated with laboratory studies. Viral or alcoholic hepatitis is the most common cause and can be suspected based on the history. Nonalcoholic steatohepatitis (NASH or fatty liver disease) is also commonly seen in the obese population [4]. Liver impairment is important due to early effects on hemostasis and the coagulability profile of the patient's blood. Coagulation studies are imperative, and precautions such as blood type and screen or even crossmatching of blood products for surgery should be taken. If signs of cirrhosis or late-stage liver disease are appreciated, the patient should be referred to a hepatologist for management prior to any elective surgical procedure.

Patients with symptoms secondary to biliary calculi should also be worked up as some surgeons will consider cholecystectomy at or following a bariatric surgical procedure. Substantial weight loss is famous for instigating formation of gallstones and biliary colic or cholecystitis.

9.6   Infectious/Immune

Patients with a known HIV infection should continue to be followed by an infectious disease specialist and continued on their antiretroviral medications. Of note, antiretroviral regimens used in HIV maintenance are not considered immunosuppressive and should not impact wound healing. Patients undergoing pharmacological antirejection regimens for organ transplants should be considered at higher risk for poor wound healing, especially if steroids are included [4]. Of note, the sleeve gastrectomy is typically preferred in these patients as there will be less effects on absorption of these lifesaving medications compared to a malabsorptive procedure such as the Roux-en-Y gastric bypass.

9.7 Hematological

History taking on every potential bariatric surgery patient will take careful note of any signs indicative of increased bleeding or hypercoagulability. Typical traits include a personal or family history of easy bruising or abnormal bleeding. Evidence of either in the history or on physical exam merit further workup. Coagulation studies are not typically ordered unless a suspicion arises. Also of note is a history of DVT or PE. Further, many patients present with pharmaco-logic anticoagulation in place for venous thromboembolism, chronic atrial fibrillation, or a history of mechanical heart valves. Warfarin is the traditional and most common anticoagulant of choice, but many newer medications with various mechanisms of action may also be encountered. A risk/benefit analysis of the patient's anticoagulation and underlying medical problem will be dis-cussed between his/her prescribing medical doctor and the surgeon. If a sub-stantial risk of complication exists, then the patient may need to be bridged from his/her chronic anticoagulant to a shorter-acting medication for the pre- and perioperative period. For example, the oral medication would be stopped 5–7 days prior to the operation (based on the half-life and pharmacokinetics), and a shorter-acting anticoagulant such as low-molecular-weight heparin would be started. This medication can then be held one day prior to the operation and restarted as soon as postoperative day zero [3]. Most bariatric surgeries do not pose a major bleeding risk, but in some instances blood products may be requested to be on hand for bleeding complications. In the super morbidly obese patient with a history of DVT or PE, a temporary inferior vena cava filter is indicated and will be removed postoperatively once full anticoagulation can be safely resumed.

9.8 Psychological

A necessary component of the preoperative workup includes psychological evalua-tion of the patient's behavioral, emotional, and developmental position in life as well as his/her expectations of the surgery and motivation for having it. Important factors that must be documented are previous attempts at weight loss (method and duration), the style of eating the patient undertakes, level of activity and involve-ment in exercise, any substance use issues, and any current life stressors. The expec-tations and goals of the patient must be asked and clearly compared against the realities of surgery. Based on the psychological background of the patient, these evaluations may be made by the surgeon, other qualified office staff, or even via consultation to an independent psychologist or psychiatrist. Some patients may be deemed unacceptable candidates for bariatric surgery if they fail the psychological evaluation. Interventions may include education and counseling as patients must understand that bariatric surgery entails lifelong behavior modification and is not a cure in and of itself.

Once selected for surgery, the patient will undergo evaluation by the anesthesiology service in regard to choice of anesthetic technique and other clinical management decisions. The American Society of Anesthesiologists system classifies patients as [4]:

I. A normal healthy patient
II. Mild systemic disease
III. Severe systemic disease which limits activity
IV. Incapacitating disease which poses a constant threat to life
V. Moribund patient who would expire within 24 h without an operation
VI. Organ procurement

Morbid obesity with a BMI greater than 40 qualifies a patient as a minimum of ASA Class III.

Considerations on the day of operation are also specific to the obese patient. Morbid obesity stands as an independent risk factor for venous thromboembolic disease. Strict adherence to a regimen designed to prevent deep vein thrombosis is mandatory. Perioperative antibiotic dosing should be adjusted appropriately to account for the increased body mass index. Finally, morbidly obese patients are at increased risk for wound infections, although this is greatly mediated in the setting of laparoscopic surgery.

In sum, the elective nature and complicated medical comorbidities common to morbidly obese patients make thorough preoperative evaluation and proper workup imperative. While every patient does not require a full laboratory and functional testing with consultation to every medical subspecialist, judicious use of these tools can make the difference between a successful bariatric operation and major morbidity and mortality.

Review Questions

1. Give the ASA class of the following patient: A 65-year-old female presenting for a laparoscopic sleeve gastrectomy with a BMI of 41, controlled hypertension, and controlled diabetes mellitus and who currently undergoes hemodialysis three days per week.

   A. I
   B. II
   C. III
   D. IV

2. Which of the following circumstances would necessitate cancelation of a planned bariatric surgical procedure on the day of operation?

   A. A morbidly obese 36-year-old female who is otherwise healthy but did not have a preoperative EKG or chest X-ray
   B. A 56-year-old male with chronic atrial fibrillation and a history of coronary stenting who has held his warfarin for five days but has continued taking clopidogrel (an antiplatelet medication)

    C. A 42-year-old female with a bedside blood glucose of 189
    D. A 60-year-old female on chronic renal replacement therapy with a potassium level of 7.2

3. Which of the following patient comorbidities would most likely disqualify him/her from undergoing bariatric surgery during the preoperative evaluation?

    A. A BMI of 90
    B. A history of daily alcohol and tobacco abuse with failure to cease
    C. Myocardial infarction with catheterization and stenting 11 months ago
    D. Severe obstructive sleep apnea requiring CPAP for sleep
    E. Poorly controlled diabetes mellitus

Answers

1. The answer is *C*. While controlled DM and hypertension qualify as mild systemic diseases and alone would qualify as an ASA class II, end-stage renal disease and morbid obesity both are considered to be severe, limiting systemic diseases, and garner an ASA III designation.
2. The answer is *D*. Hyperkalemia can represent a life-threatening electrolyte abnormality, especially in the setting of general anesthesia administration. Patients experiencing symptoms and EKG changes or with a potassium value greater than 7 should be treated immediately. Preoperative EKG, chest X-ray, and even laboratory studies are often ordered on patients but are not expressly necessary unless they have an existing condition or complaint that warrants further investigation. That being said, bariatric surgeries are done as elective procedures, and as such every effort should be made to maintain the utmost in safety. Plavix or other antiplatelet medications should be continued in patients with coronary stents, especially for the first year. Coumadin should be held at least 5 days prior to elective operations.
3. The answer is *B*. Patients who are non-compliant and or have substance abuse issues rarely do well following bariatric surgery. While the operation is helpful, continued and persistent weight loss requires ongoing lifestyle changes. Further, tobacco use is a primary risk factor for postoperative leaks, wound infections, and malnutrition. Alcohol use further worsens the nutritional status, and its continued use is a sign of poor commitment on the patient's part. The patient in choice C should be thoroughly evaluated by his cardiologist and optimized for surgery, but coronary artery disease and revascularization more than 6 weeks ago do not specifically preclude surgery. Choices A, D, and E are all indications for bariatric surgery and would be expected to improve or resolve postoperatively.

References

1. Dimick JB, Chen SL, Taheri PA et al (2004) Hospital costs associated with surgical complications: a report from the private-sector National Surgical Quality Improvement Program. J Am Coll Surg 199:531–537
2. Eagle KA, Berger PB, Calkins H et al (2002) ACC/AHA guideline update for perioperative cardiovascular evaluation for noncardiac surgery—executive summary: a report of the American College of Cardiology/American Heart Association Task Force on Practice Guidelines. J Am Coll Cardiol 39:542–553
3. Halaszynski TM, Juda R, Silverman DG (2004) Optimizing postoperative outcomes with efficient preoperative assessment and management. Crit Care Med 32:s76–s86
4. Townsend CM, Sabiston DC (2004) Sabiston textbook of surgery: the biological basis of modern surgical practice. Saunders, Philadelphia

Positioning the Bariatric Patient in the OR

10

Neha Patel and Elton Taylor

10.1 Goals of Positioning

Positioning the bariatric patient to prepare to undergo surgical intervention is an important step in preventing complications in the perioperative period. An interprofessional unit is required with the combined efforts of the physician, the surgical nursing staff, and the anesthesia staff to prepare for an uneventful procedure [1, 2]. Patient immobility is a risk factor for complications and more so in the bariatric patient. Comfort and safety with prevention of injuries are the basis for some of the positioning tactics which will be discussed. Maintaining airway and circulation and exposure of operative site also need to be taken into account when positioning the bariatric patient for continued care throughout the case.

10.2 Airway Challenges (Risk of Aspiration)

There are many challenges with regard to the anesthesia management of the bariatric patient. Excess tissue over the neck, chest, and fat pads in the oral pharynx can make access difficult. Partial airway obstruction secondary to this extra fat also leads to more difficulty with vocal cord visualization. Extra weight on the neck and chest can also lead to obstructive sleep apnea (OSA) with resulting increased rate of oxygen desaturation. Oxygenation is important for preoxygenation prior to intubation. Adequate oxygenation allows for enough time to carefully intubate the patient. Extra weight and increased gastric pressure also increase aspiration risk, and there is increased risk of damage with aspiration. One way to prevent this is to give histamine antagonists preoperatively as well as insisting a fasting state is started at midnight, the night before the procedure [3].

N. Patel, DO (✉) • E. Taylor, DO, MBA
Department of General Surgery, Rowan University, Stratford, NJ, USA
e-mail: Pateln@rowan.edu; Taylore0@rowan.edu

© Springer International Publishing Switzerland 2017
A. Loveitt et al. (eds.), *Passing the Certified Bariatric Nurses Exam*,
DOI 10.1007/978-3-319-41703-5_10

45

10.3 Cardiac/Vascular/Other Challenges

In obese patients there is increased cardiac stress at baseline from the additional body weight. There is also increased pressure on the inferior vena cava [2]. This combination can impede circulation and alter hemodynamics making it crucial that they are closely monitored during the procedure. Patients are more susceptible to increased or decreased heart rate, slowed conduction, and ischemia. Extra chest fat and tissue can also impede ECG tracing to accurately monitor the patient's rhythm [2].

Obesity, as well as the reverse Trendelenburg position (feet down), also puts patients at an increased risk for deep venous thromboses (DVTs). There is increased pressure on dependent surfaces and, in this position, the legs, increasing the risk of DVT in the legs [4]. It is extremely important that the thromboembolic device stockings are placed correctly with the stockings fitting appropriately, as to not cause a tourniquet effect, and that the stocking is smooth and not rolled up or down. Often, a patient may receive anticoagulation preoperatively.

10.4 Positioning

As mentioned above, supine and lithotomy positioning can have a detrimental effect in the operating room during a long procedure. Reverse Trendelenburg position can offset many of these challenges. This position effectively off-loads abdominal contents from the diaphragm, thus increasing functional residual capacity and pulmonary compliance and thus improving oxygenation. Footboards are placed at the patient's feet and secured to support the patient while in reverse Trendelenburg position and reduce shearing effect on the patient's skin [5].

Pressure points between the patient and the operating room table are cushioned with foam padding to prevent tissue breakdown and injury. A pillow is placed under the patient's knees to reduce lower back strain. A grounding pad is placed on the patient and metal is freed from contacting the patient's body. Arms are abducted greater than 85° from the patient's side, allowing adequate blood flow to upper extremities as well as distal IV and monitoring access to the anesthesia team (Fig. 10.1) [6]. A blanket is placed over the patient's lower extremities, and a strap is placed over the patient to secure the patient to the table. Caution must be taken not to secure the strap too tightly as this may lead to nerve injury. Slight flexion of the hips allows for increased intra-abdominal work space [7]. As mentioned above, a tourniquet effect can be easily missed during patient positioning. It is important that all gowns are removed off the patient prior to positioning. Blankets should be placed flat over the patient, taking care to free any portion that may be wrapped around or under the patient.

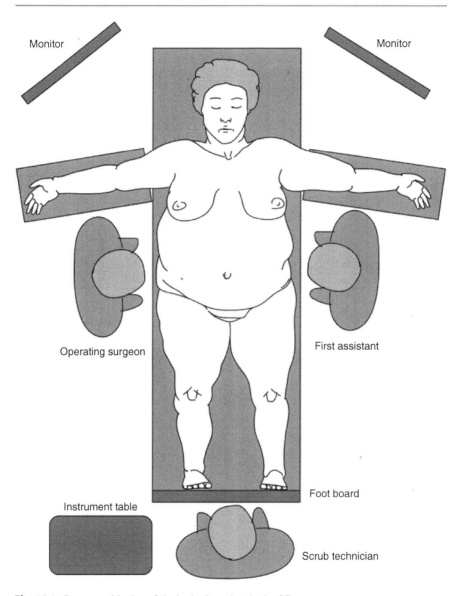

Fig. 10.1 Proper positioning of the bariatric patient in the OR

10.5   Postoperative

Postoperatively, it is important to make sure the patient is extubated easily and successfully. The anesthesia team will make sure to extubate only after a patient can follow simple commands and demonstrate good tidal volumes independently. Once the patient is extubated, they should be safely transported off the surgical table. A bariatric bed should be available as well as a bariatric sliding sheet with plenty of staff available to help transport the patient [4].

As the patient is transferred to the postanesthesia care unit (PACU), a transfer of care report should be given. All incision sites should be reassessed for integrity. All potential pressure points should also be assessed for any signs of ulceration or ecchymosis. Skin folds should be carefully examined as these can be easily missed. Intravenous fluids should be continued for additional resuscitation. Thromboembolic compression stockings should be continued. A monitor should also be attached to continue to assess for perfusion, oxygenation, and hemodynamic stability with continuous vital signs. Deep breathing and coughing should be encouraged once the patient is able to sit upright and follow more complex commands. Once this has been achieved and the patient meets discharge criteria, they will be transported to a hospital floor and continue on with phase I of the bariatric postoperative course.

Review Questions

1. What is the preferred patient position for patients undergoing bariatric surgery?

   A. Supine in Trendelenburg to allow patient higher lung volumes
   B. Supine in reverse Trendelenburg to allow patient higher lung volumes
   C. Prone in Trendelenburg to allow decreased intra-abdominal pressure
   D. Prone in reverse Trendelenburg to allow decreased intra-abdominal pressure

2. All of the following affect extubation in the bariatric patient *except*?

   A. BMI of 39
   B. Use of CPAP as an outpatient
   C. Reverse Trendelenburg positioning intraoperatively and at time of extubation
   D. Preoxygenation to SpO2 100 % prior to intubation

3. A patient just underwent a laparoscopic sleeve gastrectomy. After awakening from anesthesia, the patient complains of inability to feel their left hand. What is the most likely cause?

   A. Lack of padding at left elbow
   B. Lack of padding at left shoulder
   C. Hyperextension of patient's neck during procedure
   D. Improper placement of blood pressure cuff

4. Which of the following is the patient placed in reverse Trendelenburg at higher risk of?

A. DVT of the legs
B. Decreased lung volumes
C. Decreased oxygenation
D. Hypoglycemia

Answers

1. The answer is *B*. Bariatric surgery is most commonly performed in the supine reverse Trendelenburg position. This allows the lungs to maximally expand by taking pressure off the diaphragm, thus increasing the functional residual capacity of the lungs. Patients will oxygenate better in reverse Trendelenburg position. Trendelenburg position will increase diaphragmatic pressure, thus decreasing functional residual capacity, causing lower lung volumes and difficulty oxygenating the patient. Prone positioning allows for improved oxygenation, but is not used in bariatric surgery.

2. The answer is *D*. Airway management is important in bariatric surgery. Obese patients can provide many challenges and sometimes be very difficult to intubate and extubate; thus, proper positioning and preparation are key. Preoxygenating a patient with supplemental oxygen for a period of minutes prior to intubation allows the person intubating a longer amount of apnea time before hypoxia ensues; thus, preoxygenation affects intubation, not extubation. Of obese patients, 77 % will suffer from obstructive sleep apnea (OSA) and are treated with nocturnal continuous positive airway pressure (CPAP) to maintain oxygenation. A BMI of 39 should not prevent extubation. Maintaining a patient in reverse Trendelenburg position during extubation allows for larger lung tidal volumes and better oxygenation for extubation.

3. The answer is *B*. This patient is exhibiting symptoms of ulnar nerve palsy, likely secondary to lack of or improper padding of the left elbow as the ulnar nerve passes medially. Pressure points must be adequately padded to prevent skin injury, vascular compression, and nerve compression. Commonly padded bony pressure points include the elbows, sacrum, scapulae, and heel. Modern operating room tables have padding to cushion the entire patient, with additional padding provided with viscoelastic gel pads and foam.

4. The answer is *A*. Reverse Trendelenburg, although the ideal position for bariatric surgery, does lead to increased pressure in the lower extremities. This increased pressure leads to a higher risk of DVTs. It is extremely important that thromboembolic devices or sequential compression devices be placed and turned on prior to anesthesia induction and start of the procedure. Many times, the surgeon may order preoperative anticoagulation as well.

References

1. Fencl JL et al (2015) The bariatric patient: an overview of perioperative care. AORN J 102(2):116–131
2. Knight D, Mahajan R (2004) Patient positioning in anesthesia. Oxf J Contin Educ Anaesth Crit Care Pain 4(5):160–163
3. Kristensen MS (2010) Airway management and morbid obesity. Eur J Anesthesiol 27(11):923–927
4. Owers CE, Abbas Y, Ackroyd R et al (2012) Perioperative optimization of patients undergoing bariatric surgery. J Obes 2012:6
5. Ramos AC et al (2015) Technical aspects of laparoscopic sleeve gastrectomy. Arquivos Brasileiros de Cirurgia Digestiva 28:65–68
6. Wentzell J, Neff M (2015) The weight is over: RN first assisting techniques for laparoscopic sleeve gastrectomy. AORN J 102(2):161–180
7. Mulier JP, Dillemans B, Van Cauwenberge S (2010) Impact of the patient's body position on the intraabdominal workspace during laparoscopic surgery. Surg Endosc 24(6):1398–1402

Anesthesia in the Bariatric Patient

11

Sunny Kar

Successful surgical management of obesity requires the appropriate utilization of anesthesia; derived from the Greek roots *an* for without and *aisthēsis* for sensation. Modern surgical techniques and advances have been the direct result of anesthetic technology. Prior to the advent of the sedative, relaxing, and amnesic capacities offered, operations were limited by patient tolerance and as such had considerably higher rates of failure and complication.

As with any special population, there are challenges that come with anesthesia when applied to the bariatric patient. Due to the variation in anatomy in obese patients, attention must be directed in particular to the cardiopulmonary system. Airway management specifically is a challenge that must be adequately evaluated in the preoperative setting. Increased soft tissue in the upper thorax and neck results in limitations in movement at the atlantoaxial joint and cervical spine. Further, there are increased folds in pharyngeal soft tissue. As such, challenges should be anticipated, and having advanced airway tools such as fiber optic laryngoscopes available will alleviate such issues. The anatomical contribution extends to ventilation, with increased work of breathing due to soft tissue stresses on the chest wall.

Drug metabolism is also affected by obesity. There is an increased volume of distribution because of greater body weight, and as such loading and maintenance doses must be recalculated by the anesthesia and surgical team.

Preoperative risk assessment should take into consideration the existence of comorbidities that could be addressed, as well as experiences with previous surgery and intubation. The size of the neck diameter is a predictor of intubation difficulty [1]. Routine laboratory testing should include polysomnography, in order to institute continuous positive airway pressure in patients previously undiagnosed with obstructive sleep apnea.

S. Kar, DO
Department of General Surgery, Rowan University, Stratford, NJ, USA
e-mail: Sunnykar@gmail.com

© Springer International Publishing Switzerland 2017

51

A. Loveitt et al. (eds.), *Passing the Certified Bariatric Nurses Exam*,
DOI 10.1007/978-3-319-41703-5_11

The mechanical factors present in the preoperative arena are also to be addressed in the operating room. This includes positioning for both operative ease and induction of anesthesia. Allowing adequate access to the neck and head will greatly increase the likelihood of uncomplicated intubation. Further care should be taken to address pressure points that are subject to shear stress from the extended periods on the operating table. Establishing peripheral intravenous access in the obese patient carries its own challenges and should be anticipated and accounted for in the perioperative period. Intraoperatively, ventilation, intra-abdominal pressures, and vital signs should be closely monitored as with any surgery, but here too, there are particular nuances that are affected by body mass.

Post-procedure care is merely an extension of preoperative management. Pain control, thromboembolism prophylaxis, and encouragement of breathing exercise are mainstays of appropriate management [2]. Obese patients are especially prone to hypercoagulability, and active measures to mitigate this risk should be instituted immediately [3]. Pharmacologic control of nausea, with prevention of emesis, is exceptionally critical as it will protect the postsurgical abdomen from the shear stress of retching.

Review Questions

1. Which of the following contribute to a difficult airway in obese patients?

   A. BMI
   B. Neck circumference
   C. Cervical immobility
   D. A and B
   E. All of the above

2. What are the considerations for drug dosing in the bariatric patient?

   A. Volume of distribution
   B. Renal and hepatic function
   C. A and B only
   D. Fat solubility
   E. All of the above

3. What is the most sensitive indicator of lung function in the obese patient noted on pulmonary function tests?

   A. Tidal volume
   B. Expiratory reserve capacity
   C. Total lung capacity
   D. Dead space

4. Why are obese patients prone to rhabdomyolysis?

   A. Poor kidney function
   B. Poor fluid intake
   C. Prolonged immobility
   D. Inappropriate positioning

5. Which of the following is NOT a goal of effective anesthesia?

    A. Muscle relaxation
    B. Sedation
    C. Euphoria
    D. Amnesia

Answers

1. The answer is *E*. Cervical immobility, neck circumference, and BMI all contribute to difficulty in establishing an airway, with neck circumference having the greatest predictive value.
2. The answer is *C*. Volume of distribution is greater in obese patients, requiring higher doses of induction. Renal and hepatic metabolism are usually marginally increased as a result of increased intravascular volume, but since obese patients have an increase in mass but NOT in lean body weight, there is no compensatory increase in renal and hepatic function. While lipophilic drugs are stored longer in obese patients, there is no change in metabolism.
3. The answer is *C*. Expiratory reserve capacity has the greatest predictor of obesity affecting lung function.
4. The answer is *D*. Pressure points result in muscle breakdown and rhabdomyolysis.
5. The answer is *C*. Euphoria is not a part of anesthesia.

References

1. Brodsky JB, Lemmens HJ, Brock-Utne JG et al (2002) Morbid obesity and tracheal intubation. Anesth Analg 94:732–736
2. Yao F-SF, Savarese JJ (1998) Morbid obesity. In: Anesthesiology: problem oriented patient management. Lippincott-Raven, Philadelphia, pp 1001–1018
3. Charlebois D, Wilmoth D (2004) Critical care of patients with obesity. Crit Care Nurse 24:19–27

General Overview of the Laparoscopic Adjustable Band

12

Nidhi Khanna

The laparoscopic adjustable gastric banding (LAGB) is one of the several weight loss procedures performed in the USA today. The history of gastric banding dates back to 1978 when Dr. Wilkinson wrapped a Marlex mesh around a portion of the stomach to create a smaller gastric pouch. The first gastric banding in the USA was performed in 1980 in Texas by Dr. Molina with Dacron material [1]. Since the work of these pioneers, many technological advances have been made, and the band material is currently made from silicone. There are currently two laparoscopic adjustable bands in the market, the LAP-BAND System by Allergan and the REALIZE Band produced by Johnson & Johnson.

The preoperative work-up is similar to other types of weight loss surgery. Patients who qualify for the operation are those with a BMI >40 or BMI > 35 with comorbid conditions such as obstructive sleep apnea, diabetes, and hypertension. They must also undergo a thorough nutritional evaluation, diet education, and psychiatric evaluation prior to being considered for the operation [2].

The LAGB is classified as a restrictive procedure along with other bariatric procedures like vertical banded gastroplasty and sleeve gastrectomy (discussed in other chapters). The procedure is performed under general anesthesia. The patient is placed in reverse Trendelenburg position (head up). Five to six laparoscopic ports are placed. The angle of His (the junction between the esophagus and cardia of the stomach) is dissected circumferentially, and a tunnel is created posterior to the stomach. The band is passed under this tunnel and wrapped around the upper portion of the stomach (Fig. 12.1). This is connected to tubing and a port. The port is conveniently positioned in the subcutaneous tissue to allow for bedside access to the balloon [3].

The benefit of a LAGB is that it is a minimally invasive procedure that does not require partial removal of the stomach or diversion of the gastrointestinal tract as in

N. Khanna, DO
Department of General Surgery, Rowan University, Stratford, NJ, USA
e-mail: khannani@rowan.edu

© Springer International Publishing Switzerland 2017
A. Loveitt et al. (eds.), *Passing the Certified Bariatric Nurses Exam*,
DOI 10.1007/978-3-319-41703-5_12

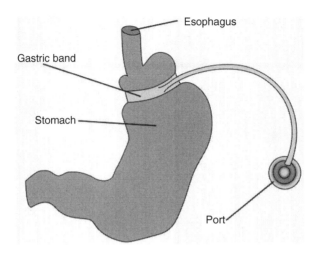

Fig. 12.1 Laparoscopic adjustable band

gastric sleeve or bypass procedures. However, patients do have to follow up with their surgeon frequently for adjustment of the band. In addition, because this is a restrictive procedure only, patients must maintain a strict diet to avoid inability to lose weight or the possibility of weight gain. Lastly, because general anesthesia is required, this surgery may not be suitable for those deemed high-risk surgical candidates.

Early complications of the lap band are food intolerance and band slippage. Nausea, vomiting, and food intolerance may require removing fluid from the band via the subcutaneous port. Late complications are band erosion, esophageal dilatation, gastric obstruction, and port or tubing problems such as infection. These complications most often lead to hospital admission and frequent reoperation [2].

Postoperative gastric band patients must have strict follow-up with their bariatric surgeon in order to track weight loss and adjust fluid in the band. Regular follow-up with a nutritionist is also important to assess caloric intake, review types of foods being consumed, address any issues related to food intolerance, etc. Patients who undergo LAGB can potentially lose up to 50 % percent of excess body weight [3].

References

1. Oria HE (1999) Gastric banding for morbid obesity. Eur J Gastroenterol Hepatol 11:105–114
2. Fady M, Brethauer SA, Schauer PR (2011) Laparoscopic surgery for severe obesity. In: Cameron's current surgical therapy. Elsevier Saunder: Philadelphia, PA, USA; p 90
3. SAGES Guidelines Committee (2008) SAGES guideline for clinical application of laparoscopic bariatric surgery. Surg Endosc 22(10):2281–2300

Laparoscopic Gastric Band: Early and Late Complications

13

Nidhi Khanna

Laparoscopic adjustable gastric banding (LAGB), although a good option for weight loss, does have its associated complications.

Early complications:

- Food intolerance
- Obstruction
- Perforation
- Venous/pulmonary thromboembolism
- Bleeding
- Infection (early or late)

Late complications:

- Band erosion
- Band slippage (early or late)
- Pouch enlargement
- Esophageal dilatation
- Port or tubing defects
- Failed weight loss

Food intolerance exhibited by nausea and vomiting is the most common early complication associated with LAGB but can also be an indication of obstruction. Obstruction occurs at an incidence of 0.5–11 % [1]. Simply adjusting the fluid in the band may help alleviate these symptoms. While adjustment may be done at

N. Khanna, DO
Department of General Surgery, Rowan University, Stratford, NJ, USA
e-mail: khannani@rowan.edu

© Springer International Publishing Switzerland 2017
A. Loveitt et al. (eds.), *Passing the Certified Bariatric Nurses Exam*,
DOI 10.1007/978-3-319-41703-5_13

the bedside, many surgeons prefer to do it under flouroscopy for ease of both the patient and the surgeon. Band slippage can also lead to obstruction and will be discussed later in the chapter. Perforation is rare and the incidence is less than 1 % [1].

Non-band-related complications are bleeding, wound infection, and venous thromboembolism (VTE). The incidence of VTE varies and is reported at less than 1 % to as high as 3.5 %. Pulmonary embolism (PE) is rare but can have an incidence as high as 1 %. Bariatric patients have several risk factors for VTE including but not limited to hypercoagulable state, venous stasis, and obesity hypoventilation syndrome. Patients undergoing obesity surgery must have aggressive prophylaxis and be monitored closely for signs and symptoms of VTE [2].

Another complication is failed weight loss. Because the LAGB is purely restrictive, this technique requires full compliance on the patient's part. If dietary restrictions are not followed and poor eating habits continue, this will lead to poor results. Furthermore, patients may be converted to a gastric sleeve or Roux-en-Y gastric bypass with good results [1].

Band erosion can occur in up to 6.8 % of cases [1]. Pressure from the band buckle or a tightly placed band can gradually erode into the stomach. Symptoms vary from epigastric pain to gastrointestinal bleeding to abscess. Endoscopy can be performed to make the diagnosis. Treatment is band removal, repair of stomach, or conversion to another procedure at another time [1] [2].

Band slippage is a rare incident occurring at a rate of 0.4–8 % [1] and can be divided into five classifications. Type I is an anterior slip where the band slips downwards on the stomach, and type II is a posterior slip where the posterior portion of the stomach slips upwards through the band. Type III is pouch enlargement (discussed in the following paragraph). Type IV is an immediate postoperative slip and type V is necrosis of the stomach associated with types I and II. This can be diagnosed with an upper gastrointestinal (UGI) series X-ray. Reoperation with band removal or re-positioning is warranted for this complication with the exception of type III [3]. Furthermore, patients can be converted to a gastric sleeve or bypass after several weeks if the gastric band is removed [1].

Increased pressure within the pouch over time can cause pouch enlargement (type III slippage). This increased pressure may be secondary to band over inflation or patient overeating. A UGI may be obtained to evaluate the degree of enlargement. Esophageal dilation can also be seen in these patients. Treatment is conservative in the majority of cases where the surgeon will completely deflate the band and modify eating habits. A UGI can be rechecked in 6 weeks to follow pouch size and most will return to normal size. If this is unsuccessful, the band may need to be removed [3].

1. All of the following are complications of gastric band except:

    A. Band erosion
    B. Gastric obstruction
    C. Port infection
    D. Bowel obstruction
    E. Band erosion

2. A patient presents to the emergency department with acute onset nausea,
    vomiting, and severe abdominal pain. The patient's vital signs are as fol-
    lows: temp 98.6, BP 140/80, and pulse 110. The patient relays a history
    of LAGB procedure 2 weeks ago. What is the most likely diagnosis?

    A. Gastric band erosion
    B. Gastroenteritis
    C. Band slippage
    D. Small bowel obstruction
    E. Gastric perforation

3. Which of the following complications can be managed conservatively
    (nonoperatively)?

    A. Gastric perforation
    B. Pouch enlargement
    C. Band erosion
    D. Port/tubing abscess

4. A patient is postoperative day 3 from a lap band procedure. On evalua-
    tion, the patient appears tachypneic and is requiring increasing amounts
    of oxygen to maintain an oxygen saturation. You note that the patient has
    not been compliant with ambulation and has been in bed since surgery.
    What is the likely diagnosis?

    A. Deep venous thrombus of the left leg
    B. Band slippage
    C. Port infection
    D. Pulmonary embolism

1. The answer is *D*. The gastric band is placed around the upper portion of
    the stomach. This procedure does not involve bowel or gastric resection.
    Therefore, bowel obstruction (D) is not a complication associated with
    this procedure. Band slippage (A), gastric obstruction (B), port infection
    (C), and band erosion (E) are all serious complications associated with
    this procedure and will likely require reoperation and band removal.

2. The answer is *C*. The most likely diagnosis in this scenario is band slippage (C) especially with acute onset of vomiting and abdominal pain in a patient with a recent LAGB placement. Gastric band erosion (A) and gastric perforation (E) are late complications associated with gastric banding. Gastroenteritis (B) is a possible diagnosis with these symptoms but less likely in a patient with recent gastric banding. Small bowel obstruction (D) is not likely because the gastric banding procedure does not involve small bowel.

3. The answer is *B*. Pouch enlargement (B) is a type III slippage associated with increased pressure in the stomach proximal to the band. This is usually treated by reducing fluid in the band and treating symptoms of reflux and nausea that may be present. Gastric perforation (A), band erosion (C), and port/tubing abscess (D) are all treated with reoperation and removal of the band apparatus.

4. The answer is D. This patient is displaying classic signs of an acute pulmonary embolism (D). This goes along with the patient's history of remaining in bed and not ambulating postoperatively. This is a serious postoperative complication of bariatric surgery. The bariatric team should work together to encourage and ensure that patients are out of bed and mobile to prevent VTE complications. DVT (A), band slippage (B), and port infection (C) would not present with the classic symptoms of tachypnea and hypoxia which are associated with pulmonary embolus.

References

1. Brethauer SA et al (2014) Systematic review on reoperative bariatric surgery American Society for Metabolic and Bariatric Surgery Revision Taskforce. Surg Obes Relat Dis 10:952–972
2. Jamal MH et al (2015) Thromboembolic events in bariatric surgery: a large multi-institutional referral center experience. Surg Endosc 29:376–380
3. Eid I et al (2011) Complications associated with adjustable gastric banding for morbid obesity: a surgeon's guide. Can J Surg 54(1):61–66

Laparoscopic Gastric Band: Pros and Cons

14

Nidhi Khanna

There are several positive and negative aspects associated with the laparoscopic adjustable gastric band (LAGB) listed below:

14.1 Pros

- It is a minimally invasive procedure.
- Shorter hospital stay.
- Does not require partial removal of the stomach or diversion of the gastrointestinal tract.
- Purely restrictive, therefore does not cause malabsorption.
- The only procedure that allows for outpatient adjustments after surgery.
- Demonstrates improvement in obesity-related comorbidities.
- Can be applied to obese adolescents.

14.2 Cons

- Strict diet and lifestyle modifications are required to achieve and maintain weight loss.
- Less effective weight loss than other bariatric procedures.
- May require revision or conversion to another weight loss procedure.

Let's expand on these further.

Almost all surgery for obesity is now performed laparoscopically through several small incisions making it minimally invasive. However, the LAGB has shown to

N. Khanna, DO
Department of General Surgery, Rowan University, Stratford, NJ, USA
e-mail: khannani@rowan.edu

© Springer International Publishing Switzerland 2017
A. Loveitt et al. (eds.), *Passing the Certified Bariatric Nurses Exam*,
DOI 10.1007/978-3-319-41703-5_14

impart a shorter hospital stay and shorter operative time than other minimally invasive weight loss procedures [1].

Procedures can be divided into restrictive and malabsorptive. The benefit of LAGB is that it does not require diversion of the gastrointestinal tract like laparoscopic Roux-en-Y gastric bypass or removal of a portion of the stomach like laparoscopic sleeve gastrectomy. Furthermore, the LAGB is considered a purely restrictive procedure in which patients are less likely to have malabsorption [2].

The LAGB is unique in that the band has an inflatable balloon attached to a subcutaneous port. This allows for outpatient adjustments in band volume without having to hospitalize the patient. In this way, patient weight loss can be tailored [3].

Like other weight loss procedures, patients will have an improvement in obesity-related comorbid conditions like diabetes, hypertension, and hyperlipidemia. Approximately two-thirds of patients with diabetes can achieve better glucose control or complete resolution of diabetes after LAGB. One study showed improvement in hypertension in up to 80 % of their subjects, with 55 % no longer requiring any anti-hypertensive medications. Furthermore, the LAGB has had a positive impact on illnesses like obstructive sleep apnea, gastroesophageal reflux disease, and asthma [4].

There are various criteria that need to be met prior to undertaking bariatric surgery. The majority of procedures today are only performed in adults who have a BMI > 35 with comorbid conditions or those with BMI > 40. Furthermore, this procedure is being performed in obese adolescents and has shown positive results similar to adult studies [5, 6].

In post-gastric band, patients are required to have a lifelong follow-up with their surgeon and a close follow-up with a dietitian. Lifestyle and diet modifications are integral parts of success with LAGB and maintenance of weight loss [3].

Patients can achieve between 34.7 and 53.3 % of EBW in 1 year. However, multiple studies have shown non-LAGB procedures such as gastric sleeve and Roux-en-Y gastric bypass to have superior weight loss [1].

Review Questions

1. Which of the following is a benefit of laparoscopic gastric banding compared to other weight loss procedures?

   A. Adjustable for weight loss
   B. Does not cause malabsorption
   C. Leaves gross anatomy intact
   D. All of the above

2. Which of the following patients is a good a candidate for lap band?

   A. A patient who cannot dedicate time to exercise
   B. A patient who has high cardiovascular risk with a BMI of 35
   C. A patient who has poor eating habits
   D. A patient who is able to follow up regularly

3. Which of the following laparoscopic procedures is only a restrictive weight loss surgery?

   A. Sleeve gastrectomy
   B. Roux-en-Y gastric bypass
   C. Laparoscopic gastric band
   D. Jejunal-ileal bypass
   E. None of the above

4. All of the following are the components of the gastric banding device except

   A. Subcutaneous port
   B. Port tubing
   C. Inflatable band
   D. Balloon implant
   E. None of the above

5. Which of the following is an appropriate patient for weight loss surgery?

   A. A 55-year-old healthy female with a BMI of 28
   B. A 25-year-old male with a BMI of 30, history of diabetes, and no attempt at exercising or dietary modification
   C. A 40-year-old male with a BMI of 37, hypertension, and sleep apnea
   D. A 37-year-old female with a BMI of 40 who has missed several pre-operative appointments
   E. A 60-year-old female with a BMI of 33, history of alcohol dependence, and diabetes

Answers

1. The answer is *D*. The benefits of laparoscopic gastric banding are multifold and make it an attractive option for weight loss. The band is adjustable in an outpatient setting, allowing for tailored weight loss (A), it does not remove a portion of the stomach (C), and, therefore, it does not cause malabsorption (B).
2. The answer is D. Patient selection is important prior to undertaking any bariatric procedure. Patients must be able to follow up regularly, adhere to a strict diet, and make lifestyle modifications. Those who cannot spend time to exercise (A) and have poor eating habits that cannot follow dietary restrictions (C) are not good candidates for the operation. In addition, patients who cannot undergo general anesthesia because they are at high risk (B) are excluded.
3. The answer is C. Weight loss surgery can be divided into two categories, restrictive and malabsorptive procedures. Choice C, gastric band does not remove a portion of the stomach or alter normal anatomy. This is why it is only a restrictive procedure. Ingested food is limited which allows

for more frequent meal intake, less caloric intake, and weight loss. In contrast to this, choices A, B, and D are all categorized as malabsorptive procedures.

4. The answer is D. A subcutaneous port (A), port tubing (B), and inflatable band (C) are all parts of the gastric banding device. The inflatable band is placed around the upper portion of the stomach and is connected to the band tubing. The tubing is brought out through the anterior abdominal wall, tunneled in the subcutaneous tissues, and attached to the port. The port is sutured under the skin in the subcutaneous tissues. Choice D, the balloon implant is not part of the banding apparatus.

5. The answer is B. It is important to know how to choose the appropriate patient for bariatric surgery. A BMI of 30 with comorbid conditions such as diabetes, obstructive sleep apnea, and hypertension and a BMI of 40 with no associated conditions are general criteria for weight loss surgery. In addition to this, patients must be compliant (D), undergo a psychiatric and nutritional workup, and have tried diet and exercise modifications to lose weight (B). Patients with drug or alcohol dependence are also excluded from undergoing surgery (E).

References

1. Chakravarty PD et al (2012) Review: comparison of laparoscopic adjustable gastric banding (LAGB) with other bariatric procedures; a systematic review of the randomised controlled trials. Surgeon 10:172–192
2. Bal B, Finelli F, Shope T, Koch T (2012) Nutritional deficiencies after bariatric surgery. Nat Rev Endocrinol 8(9):544–556
3. Favretti F et al (2002) Patient management after LAP-BAND placement. Am J Surg 184:38s–41s
4. Dixon JB et al (2002) Changes in comorbidities and improvements in quality of life after LAP-BAND placement. Am J Surg 184:51s–54s
5. Schmitt F et al (2016) Laparoscopic adjustable gastric banding in adolescents: results at two years including psychosocial aspects. J Pediatr Surg 51(3):403–408
6. Zitsman JL et al (2015) Adolescent laparoscopic adjustable gastric banding (LAGB): prospective results in 137 patients followed for 3 years. Surg Obes Relat Dis 11(1):101–109

General Overview of the Laparoscopic Sleeve Gastrectomy

15

Andrew Loveitt

The laparoscopic sleeve gastrectomy (LSG), or "lap sleeve," is the most recent addition to the commonly performed metabolic surgeries. The procedure was first described in 1993 as a part of the biliopancreatic diversion and subsequently began to be employed as the first part of a staged duodenal switch in the 2000s. Soon it was recognized that results from the sleeve gastrectomy alone were adequate for many patients, and the sleeve gastrectomy is now the fastest growing segment of bariatric surgery [1].

The sleeve gastrectomy is considered primarily a restrictive technique; however, there is still ongoing research involving hormonal effects, with alterations of ghrelin production being cited most often. These factors produce excellent outcomes. Patients can expect to lose up to 75 % of excess body weight with a reduction in comorbidities ranging from diabetes mellitus to hypertension within the first year after surgery.

While technique will vary slightly by surgeon, the procedure begins with introduction of the laparoscope into the abdomen. After the introduction of additional ports (typically five total) and a liver retractor, the greater omentum and short gastric vessels are freed from the stomach using an energy device. Next, starting proximal to the pylorus, a linear staple line is created toward the angle of His. This frees the greater curvature of the stomach and creates the sleeve gastrectomy. Total operating time is in the range of 1–2 h.

Postoperatively, most patients are placed on a med-surg floor with telemetry monitoring. Typically patients are kept NPO on the date of surgery, their pain and nausea controlled with IV medications, and they are encouraged to be as ambulatory as possible. On postoperative day 1, many surgeons elect to perform a gastrografin swallow. This study helps to assess the anatomy of the gastric pouch as well as evaluate for leaks. The patient will be started on a bariatric stage 1 diet (clear

A. Loveitt, DO
Department of General Surgery, Rowan University, Stratford, NJ, USA
e-mail: Loveitan@rowan.edu

© Springer International Publishing Switzerland 2017   65
A. Loveitt et al. (eds.), *Passing the Certified Bariatric Nurses Exam*,
DOI 10.1007/978-3-319-41703-5_15

liquids). With adequate pain control and motivation, most patients are discharged home on postoperative day 1 or 2.

Perhaps the most important aspect of the patient's stay is a safe discharge. The LSG leads to immediate hormonal effects making the cessation of many diabetic and antihypertensive medications possible. Most notably, diuretics are typically held to avoid dehydration as the patient is expected to have decreased fluid intake. The patient will also be discharged on oral pain medication (most commonly dilaudid for its small pill size) and antiemetics. While there is no consensus, many surgeons discharge their bariatric patients on low molecular weight heparin as well [2].

While the LSG is a safe procedure, complications can and do occur. The nurse is often the first to notice worrisome signs including tachycardia, intractable vomiting, drop in hemoglobin, and rising creatinine. The most feared complication of the sleeve gastrectomy is a staple-line leak. Other complications include staple-line bleeding and stricture, torsion, and venous thromboembolism.

Postoperative follow-up generally consists of visits at 2 weeks, 1, 3, 6, and 12 months, and then yearly thereafter. It is generally recommended that patients remain on multivitamins as well as B12, Vitamin D, and iron supplementation for life [3]. Long-term outcomes following sleeve gastrectomy are still being studied; however, it does appear to be a durable procedure with percentage of excess weight loss being greater than 50 % at 5 or more years [4].

References

1. Buchwald H (2014) The evolution of metabolic/bariatric surgery. Obes Surg 24(8):1126–1135
2. Jamal M, Cocelles R, Shimizu H et al (2015) Thromboembolic events in bariatric surgery: a large multi-institutional referral center experience. Surg Endosc 29:376–380
3. Taylor D, Lenhard MJ, Synder-Marlowe G (2010) Nutrition care for patients undergoing laparoscopic sleeve gastrectomy for weight loss. J Am Diet Assoc 110(4):600–660
4. Diamantis T, Apostolou K, Alexandrou A et al (2014) Review of long-term weight loss results after laparoscopic sleeve gastrectomy. Surg Obes Relat Dis 10(1):177–183

Laparoscopic Sleeve Gastrectomy: Pros and Cons

16

Andrew Loveitt

The laparoscopic sleeve gastrectomy (LSG) has now become the most frequently performed weight-loss procedure in the world. Most consider the laparoscopic Roux-en-Y gastric bypass (LRYGB) the "gold standard" weight-loss procedure; however, there is argument that the LSG is the new standard as there are many positives and few disadvantages [1].

16.1 Pros

- Similar weight loss to the LRYGB.
- Control of medical comorbidities including diabetes is outstanding.
- No malabsorption making nutritional deficiencies/anemia less frequent.
- Reliable absorption of life-sustaining medications (HIV, transplant, antiseizure, antipsychotic).
- Hormonal influences may reduce appetite.
- Less technically challenging procedure.
- Low overall rate of complications.
- There is no anastomosis eliminating the risk of ulcer formation and internal hernias.
- Can be used on the super obese as the first stage of a two-stage procedure.
- Durable procedure.

A. Loveitt, DO
Department of General Surgery, Rowan University, Stratford, NJ, USA
e-mail: Loveitan@rowan.edu

© Springer International Publishing Switzerland 2017
A. Loveitt et al. (eds.), *Passing the Certified Bariatric Nurses Exam*,
DOI 10.1007/978-3-319-41703-5_16

16.2   Cons

- Permanent distortion of the anatomy.
- Can increase reflux and contraindicated in Barrett's esophagus.
- The long staple line can lead to complications.

Let's look at each in detail.

There are two outcomes which should be evaluated with any weight-loss procedure – excess weight loss (EWL) and reduction in medical comorbidities. LSG has been cited as providing superior weight loss to the laparoscopic adjustable gastric band (LAGB) (EWL 66% vs. 48%) [2]. Approximately 66–80% of patients can expect complete remission of type II diabetes, hypertension, and hyperlipidemia with an even higher percentage experiencing partial remission [2]. This can be compared to the 70–80% EWL and remission of comorbidities seen in the LRYGB [3].

Fifty-seven percent of morbidly obese individuals will have some form of nutritional deficiency preoperatively [4]. In this already malnourished population, the use of malabsorptive procedures (LRYGB and duodenal switch) can lead to increased deficiencies postoperatively. Nutritional deficiencies can occur over the short and long term in up to 35% of patients undergoing a malabsorptive procedure. Vitamins A, B1, B6, B12, and D3 and macronutrients such as protein and micronutrients including zinc and iron are most commonly affected [4, 5]. While patients undergoing LSG can still experience nutritional deficiencies (specifically in protein), the overall rate is lower [4, 6].

Sleeve gastrectomy has been associated with significant hormonal effects. Most commonly implicated are more rapid gastric emptying, increase in postprandial cholecystokinin and glucagon-like peptide-1 concentrations, and reduced ghrelin release [7]. Together these have been implicated in increased satiety and weight loss as well as improved glucose metabolism.

The LSG is generally considered to be a less technically challenging procedure than the LRYGB. Operative times vary by surgeon, but studies have found the operative time for an LSG (82–101 min) to be significantly less than for the LRYGB (98–133 min) [8–10]. The overall rate of morbidity and mortality of the LSG has been found to be 5.2% and 0.4%, respectively [8]. This falls between that of the LAGB and the RNYGB. Most significant complications from the LSG occur as leaks or bleeding along the staple line created.

As previously discussed, the LSG was initially intended as the first stage of a staged procedure. The shorter operative time allows it to be safely performed on sicker patients with higher BMIs. While patients and their physicians are overwhelmingly pleased with initial outcomes, conversion to a second stage (RNYGB or DS) is still performed in approximately 2.2% of patients to improve weight loss or reduce GERD symptoms [8].

There were initially concerns about the long-term durability of weight loss with the LSG. A recent review cited %EWL 62.3%, 53.8%, 43%, and 54.8% at 5, 6, 7, and 8 or more years after LSG, respectively [11]. Multiple other studies have demonstrated %EWL at 5 years to be around 60%, and in most studies, it was not significantly different than LRYGB [2, 11]. The 5-year results have shown both LSG and

LRYGB to each have a sustained effect on medical comorbidities. Most analyses find a slightly more robust improvement in type II diabetes with the LRYGB [9].

Barrett's esophagus is an intestinal metaplasia of the esophagus and is a major risk factor for the development of esophageal adenocarcinoma. It is a result of long-term exposure of the esophagus to gastric acids. 50–70 % of patients undergoing bariatric surgery have symptoms of gastroesophageal reflux disease (GERD), and a hiatal hernia is present in 15 % [12]. Most studies find continued or even worsening GERD following LSG [1]. In comparison, LRYGB resolves GERD in the majority of cases [13]. Expert consensus is that the presence of severe GERD or Barrett's esophagus is an absolute contraindication to sleeve gastrectomy [14].

Review Questions

1. Approximately what percentage of patients undergoing a laparoscopic sleeve gastrectomy can expect to have remission of their type II diabetes?

    A. The LSG has no effect on type II diabetes.
    B. Patients can expect their blood sugar to be better controlled, but all will still require medications.
    C. 10–30 % of patients will experience remission.
    D. 60–80 % will experience remission.
    E. 100 % will experience remission.

2. The most common source of major postoperative bleeding after a laparoscopic sleeve gastrectomy is a result of:

    A. The long staple line created when resecting the stomach
    B. The anastomosis between the stomach and the jejunum
    C. The anastomosis between the jejunum and jejunum
    D. The laparoscopic port sites as they are difficult to close in the morbidly obese
    E. The esophagus after performing an intraoperative endoscopy

3. Which of the following is considered a contraindication to laparoscopic sleeve gastrectomy?

    A. BMI >60
    B. History of GERD
    C. History of Barrett's esophagus
    D. History of vitamin D deficiency
    E. BMI of 35

4. What percentage of excess weight loss can a patient expect to maintain 5 years after a laparoscopic sleeve gastrectomy?

    A. 30–40 %
    B. 40–50 %
    C. 50–70 %
    D. 70–90 %
    E. 90–100 %

5. Which of the following is true regarding the laparoscopic sleeve gastrectomy?

    A. Although it is gaining popularity, it is still the third most commonly performed weight-loss surgery in the USA.
    B. Patients with reflux symptoms are encouraged to pursue an LSG as symptoms will typically resolve postoperatively.
    C. A decrease in postprandial glucagon-like peptide-1 secretion has been implicated in increasing satiety after LSG.
    D. Once an LSG has been performed, the patient can be reverted to their natural anatomy if desired.
    E. Once an LSG has been performed, the patient can be converted to another form of weight-loss surgery if desired.

Answers

1. The answer is *D*. Although the number varies slightly between publications, in general 60–80 % of patients can expect total resolution of their type II diabetes after having an LSG.
2. The answer is *A*. Although bleeding can occur anywhere within the operative field, the best answer choice here is from along the staple line. Other sources of major bleeding can occur from omental vessels as well as the spleen. A patient having an LSG would not have an anastomosis at either the stomach or jejunum. Significant bleeding from the port sites or esophagus is rare.
3. The answer is *C*. The major contraindication to LSG is Barrett's esophagus. The presence of reflux itself is not a contraindication although many surgeons may suggest a LRYGB in this case. LSG is the preferred procedure in the super obese but can also be performed in patients with a BMI of 35 or greater if they have at least two obesity-related comorbidities. Many bariatric patients have a history of vitamin deficiencies and will require supplements perioperatively.
4. The answer is C. After an LSG, patients can expect to maintain 50–70 % of excess weight loss at 5 years.
5. The answer is E. The LSG is unique in that it can be used as the initial stage of a two-stage procedure. This technique was originally developed for the super obese patient with multiple comorbidities. The LSG is now the most commonly performed weight-loss procedure in the USA followed by LRYGB and LAGB. An increase in postprandial GLP-1 leads to greater satiety. The LSG requires excising a large portion of the stomach, this is removed from the patient's body, and there is no way to revert back.

References

1. Buwen J, Kammerer M, Beekley A et al (2015) Laparoscopic sleeve gastrectomy: the rightful gold standard weight loss surgery procedure. Surg Obes Relat Dis 11(6):1383–1385
2. A. C. I. Committee (2012) Updated position statement on sleeve gastrectomy as a bariatric procedure. Surg Obes Relat Dis 8:e21–e26
3. Lamond K, Anne L (2014) Morbid obesity. In: Current surgical therapy, 11th edn. Elsevier, Philadelphia
4. Gehrer S, Kern B, Peters T, Christoffel-Courtin C, Peterli R (2010) Fewer nutrient deficiencies after laparoscopic sleeve gastrectomy (LSG) than after laparoscopic Roux-Y-gastric bypass (LRYGB) – a prospective study. Obes Surg 20(4):447–453
5. Bal B, Finelli F, Shope T, Koch T (2012) Nutritional deficiencies after bariatric surgery. Nat Rev Endocrinol 8(9):544–556
6. Verger E, Aron-Wisnesky J, Carlota Dao M et al (2016) Micronutrient and protein deficiencies after gastric bypass and sleeve gastrectomy: a 1-year follow-up. Obes Surg 26(4):785–796
7. Mans E, Serra-Prat M, Palomera E et al (2015) Sleeve gastrectomy effects on hunger, satiation and gastrointestinal hormone and motility responses after a liquid meal test. Am J Clin Nutr 102(3):540–547
8. Deital M, Gagner M, Erickson A et al (2011) Third International Summit: current status of sleeve gastrectomy. Surg Obes Relat Dis 7:749–759
9. Zhang Y, Zhao H, Cao Z et al (2014) A randomized clinical trial of laparoscopic Roux-en-Y gastric bypass and sleeve gastrectomy for the treatment of morbid obesity in China: a 5-year outcome. Obes Surg 24(10):1617–1624
10. Young M, Gebhart A, Phelen M et al (2015) Use and outcomes of laparoscopic sleeve gastrectomy vs laparoscopic gastric bypass: analysis of the American College of Surgeons NSQIP. J Am Coll Surg 220(5):880–885
11. Li JF, Lai DD, Lin ZH et al (2014) Comparison of the long-term results of Roux-en-Y gastric bypass and sleeve gastrectomy for morbid obesity: a systematic review and meta-analysis of randomized and nonrandomized trials. Surg Laparos Endosc Percutan Tech 24(1):1–11
12. Melissas J, Braghetto I, Molina J et al (2015) Gastroesophageal reflux disease and sleeve gastrectomy. Obes Surg 25:2430–2435
13. DuPree C, Blair K, Steele S, Martin M (2014) Laparoscopic sleeve gastrectomy in patients with preexisting gastroesophageal reflux disease: a national analysis. JAMA Surg 149(4):328–334
14. Gagner M (2016) Is sleeve gastrectomy always an absolute contraindication in patients with Barrett's? Obes Surg 26(4):715–717

Laparoscopic Sleeve Gastrectomy: The Procedure

17

Andrew Loveitt

The premise of the laparoscopic sleeve gastrectomy (LSG) is simple. Using a linear stapler, a vertical tube of stomach is created, therefore restricting the oral intake of the patient. In truth, the LSG has multiple hormonal effects as well. The operative steps are simple in concept, but many nuances are present. Technique varies by surgeon, but the procedure can be thought of as four discrete sections: access and exposure, resection of omental attachments to the greater curvature, resection of the stomach, and finally leak testing and closure.

17.1 Access and Exposure

The procedure begins with the patient in supine position with both arms out. The surgeon stands on the patient's right and assistant(s) to the left. Access to the bariatric abdomen can be difficult due to the excess adipose tissue. This can be further complicated by previous operations. Options for initial access and establishment of pneumoperitoneum include the use of the Veress needle (a blunt-tipped, spring-loaded needle), insertion of a 5 mm trochar under direct visualization, and the Hasson (cutdown) technique [1]. Once access has been confirmed, the abdomen is insufflated to 15 mmHg using CO_2 gas. Additional ports are then placed under direct visualization of the laparoscope. Typically, a total of 5–6 ports will be placed in the upper abdomen, at least one being a 12 mm port which is required for the stapler. The left lobe of the liver overlies the upper stomach and gastroesophageal junction necessitating a liver retractor to be placed for adequate exposure throughout the procedure. Finally, the patient is placed in steep reverse Trendelenburg (feet down) position to allow other intra-abdominal contents to fall away from the operative field.

A. Loveitt, DO
Department of General Surgery, Rowan University, Stratford, NJ, USA
e-mail: Loveitan@rowan.edu

© Springer International Publishing Switzerland 2017 73
A. Loveitt et al. (eds.), *Passing the Certified Bariatric Nurses Exam*,
DOI 10.1007/978-3-319-41703-5_17

17.2   Mobilization of the Greater Curvature
from the Omentum and Short Gastric Vessels

The greater curvature (or inferior border) of the stomach runs from the pylorus to the angle of His (junction of the most superior part of the stomach and esophagus). The greater omentum is attached to the stomach along this curve. Additionally, there are vessels running between the spleen and the stomach which must be divided. This dissection begins 2–8 cm from the pylorus and carries upward until the angle of His [2]. It is typically carried out using an energy device. When nearing the angle of His, one must pay particular attention to not damage the spleen.

17.3   Resection of the Stomach

An esophageal bougie (calibrated tube) is placed. Size is controversial and can range from 24 Fr to 48 Fr (with larger numbers indicating a larger diameter) depending on the surgeon [1, 2]. After assuring all other tubes are removed from the stomach, a linear stapler is then used to create the gastric tube along the length of the bougie starting near the pylorus and traveling toward the angle of His (Fig. 17.1). One must pay particular attention toward the superior aspect of the staple line to reduce any posterior redundancy of the stomach before firing the stapler. Failure to do so can lead to spiraling. The thickness of a stapler load corresponds to its color, and the surgeon will ask for different colored loads depending on the perceived thickness of the stomach. Typically, the first several firings of the stapler will require the thickest loads. On average, six 60 mm stapler loads will be used in total [2]. Once completed, the resected stomach is removed from the abdomen. There are various ways to reinforce the staple line including oversewing, fibrin glues, and reinforcement materials.

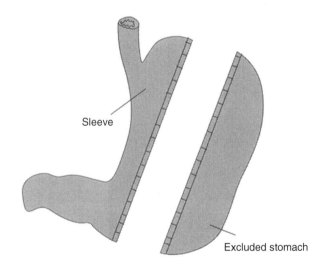

Sleeve

Fig. 17.1 Sleeve gastrectomy. The excluded stomach will be removed and discarded

Excluded stomach

17.4 Leak Testing and Closure

Once resection is complete, the staple line is inspected for defects and bleeding. Any bleeding should be controlled with surgical clips or suture as opposed to an energy source. The use of energy here could lead to thermal injury and delayed perforation. Most surgeons will then test the staple line's integrity further using one of various methods. Commonly, the staple line will be submerged in irrigant, and an endoscope will be used to inflate the stomach. If air bubbles are seen, then a leak is present. An alternate method is the instillation of methylene blue dye via an oral gastric tube [2].

Some surgeons elect to leave a closed suction (Jackson-Pratt) drain along the staple line to aid in the diagnosis of leaks or hemorrhage. This practice has largely been abandoned as studies have revealed drains indeed do not facilitate the detection of leak or bleeding [3].

Once the surgeon is satisfied with the procedure, attention is turned toward closure. All laparoscopic ports greater than 5 mm should be closed at the fascial level. The CO2 is allowed to escape from the abdomen, the patient is returned to neutral position, and the skin is closed using absorbable suture and skin sealant.

Review Questions

1. What gas is typically used to insufflate the abdomen during laparoscopic procedures?

   A. Helium
   B. Compressed room air
   C. Carbon dioxide
   D. Carbon monoxide

2. Which of the following has the steps performed during a laparoscopic sleeve gastrectomy in the proper order?

   A. Anduction of anesthesia, takedown of the short gastric vessels, placement of the liver retractor, and resection of the stomach
   B. Placing the patient in reverse Trendelenburg position, takedown of the short gastric vessels, bougie placement, and resection of the stomach
   C. Placing the patient in reverse Trendelenburg position, takedown of the splenic vessels, bougie placement, and resection of the stomach
   D. Veress needle insertion, resection of the stomach, takedown of the short gastric vessels, and closure of the fascia at the 5 mm port sites

3. Which is the preferred method of entry into the abdomen for a laparoscopic sleeve gastrectomy?

   A. Hasson (cutdown) technique.
   B. Veress needle.
   C. Direct visual entry using a laparoscopic trochar.
   D. All of the above are acceptable means of entry.

4. Why is the reverse Trendelenburg (feet down) position preferred during laparoscopic sleeve gastrectomy?

   A. It increases exposure by allowing intra-abdominal contents to fall toward the feet.
   B. It increases blood return to the heart through the assistance of gravity.
   C. It creates tension on the stomach making the dissection easier.
   D. This is not the preferred position; the patient should be placed in Trendelenburg (feet up).

5. While inspecting the staple line, the surgeon notices a brisk bleeder. Which of the following would be acceptable instruments to hand him (multiple answers may be correct)?

   A. The LigaSure device
   B. A laparoscopic needle driver loaded with 0-Vicryl suture
   C. The harmonic scalpel
   D. Bovie electrocautery
   E. Laparoscopic clip applier

Answers

1. The answer is *C*. Carbon dioxide (CO_2) is the gas typically used in laparoscopy. It is an inert gas that is a normal end product of metabolism. It rapidly diffuses into the bloodstream where it can then be removed through respiration. Although helium and room air have been used experimentally, they are not the most common options.

2. The answer is *B*. A is incorrect because the liver retractor would be placed during the first part of the procedure to aid in exposure throughout the case. C is incorrect because one wants to avoid damaging the *splenic* vessels while dissecting the greater curvature of the stomach. D is incorrect because the short gastric vessels should be divided before resecting the stomach, and also, most surgeons do not close the fascia of 5 mm port sites.

3. The answer is *D*. Method of entry is based on surgeon preference, and all of the above are acceptable.

4. The answer is *A*. The reverse Trendelenburg position is preferred to increase exposure for the surgeon. The blood return is actually *worsened* in reverse Trendelenburg, and communication with the anesthesia team is paramount during positioning. Tension on the stomach is created by the surgeon and their assistant; positioning plays a minimal role.

5. The answer is *B* and *E*. When handling the staple line and any portion of the stomach which will remain, the surgeon must avoid the use of thermal energy as this can lead to thermal injury, eventual necrosis, and leakage.

References

1. Buchwald H (2012) Sleeve gastrectomy. In: Buchwald's atlas of metabolic & bariatric surgical techniques. Elsevier, Philadelphia, PA, pp 211–227
2. Zeni T (2009) Minimally invasive sleeve gastrectomy. In: Atlas of minimally invasive surgery. Elsevier, Philadephia, PA, pp 75–77
3. Albanopoulos K, Alevizos L, Linardoutsos D et al (2011) Routine abdominal drains after laparoscopic sleeve gastrectomy: a retrospective review of 353 patients. Obes Surg 21(6):687–691

Laparoscopic Sleeve Gastrectomy: Recognizing and Treating Complications

18

Andrew Loveitt

The overall rate of serious morbidity from the laparoscopic sleeve gastrectomy (LSG) is 3.8%, and 30-day mortality rate is 0.1% [1]. Complications unique to LSG include staple line leaks and stricture or obstruction of the gastric lumen. The bedside nurse must also be vigilant for complications that can present in all surgical patients including bleeding, DVT/PE, and infectious processes.

18.1 Staple Line Leaks

Inherent to LSG is the creation of a long staple line to form the gastric pouch. Gastric leakage from this staple line can be a life-threatening complication which occurs in 1–3% of LSG and is the most common cause of major morbidity and mortality [2, 3]. To prevent this complication, surgeons have attempted to reinforce the staple line either through the use of a buttressing material, through application of sealants, or by oversewing. There is no consensus on the preferred technique, and this seems to have a larger effect on bleeding than leakage [4]. Leaks can be classified as mechanical (stapler misfire, direct tissue injury) which present within 2 days of surgery or ischemic which appear 5–6 days postoperatively. Late leaks have been noted up to 16 months after surgery [4].

From a nursing perspective, the most important aspect is early recognition. Most agree that tachycardia, specifically a HR >120, is the most important and constant indication of a leak. This is often accompanied by acute (early) or more chronic (late) abdominal pain and fevers. Although an elevated WBC count or CRP may be present, this is difficult to interpret in the presence of a recent surgery [4]. When a leak is suspected, CT scan with IV and PO water-soluble contrast is the best noninvasive test [3].

A. Loveitt, DO
Department of General Surgery, Rowan University, Stratford, NJ, USA
e-mail: Loveitan@rowan.edu

© Springer International Publishing Switzerland 2017
A. Loveitt et al. (eds.), *Passing the Certified Bariatric Nurses Exam*,
DOI 10.1007/978-3-319-41703-5_18

There is no consensus on the management of postoperative leaks. However, the first question that must be asked is if the patient is stable or unstable. If unstable, the answer is to return to the OR for washout and drainage. If stable, the management becomes more complicated. Typically conservative approaches are favored including IV hydration, NPO, PPIs, parenteral nutrition, percutaneous drainage, and broad-spectrum antibiotics and antifungals. If there is a persistent leak (2 weeks) despite conservative management, endoscopic therapies including clipping, application of fibrin glue, and stenting can be attempted. If all else fails, the patient will need a revisional surgery which could include conversion to a Roux-en-Y gastric bypass or even a total gastrectomy with esophageal-jejunal anastomosis [3, 4].

18.2 Bleeding

Bleeding requiring transfusion occurs in 0.65 % of patients following a LSG, and bleeding from the staple line itself is thought to occur in 1–2 % of patients [1, 2]. While a relatively uncommon complication, bleeding can present insidiously or as a major hemorrhage requiring rapid intervention. There are many potential bleeding sites after an LSG including the gastric staple line, gastric and omental vessels, lacerations to the liver or spleen, and trochar sites. The best treatment for bleeding is prevention through careful dissection and reinforcement of the staple line [5]. Bleeding typically presents on postoperative day zero or one. It is detected clinically in the majority of cases by tachycardia, hypotension, and decreased urine output. Bloody vomiting or dark stools may occur [6]. A drop in hemoglobin may also be present but should not be relied on for diagnosis.

Stable patients can be treated conservatively with cessation of blood thinners, transfusion, and close monitoring. Endoscopic evaluation may also be beneficial. If the patient is unstable or the bleeding is persistent, they should be taken back to the OR for exploration, washout, and control of bleeding which can typically be accomplished laparoscopically.

18.3 Venous Thromboembolism (VTE)

The risk of pulmonary embolism (PE) and deep vein thrombosis (DVT) after any bariatric surgery is less than 0.5 %. Procedure type does appear to significantly impact the incidence of VTE. Duodenal switch carries the highest risk, while LSG and laparoscopic adjustable band are safest [7]. The majority of events occur after discharge from the hospital. While there is a low incidence of PE, this is a significant event resulting in 17–33 % of all postbariatric mortalities [8].

18.4 Infections

Wound infections, intra-abdominal abscess, and pneumonia all occur in less than 1 % of patients undergoing LSG [1]. Careful clinical exam is paramount in the identification of these complications. Erythema or drainage from wounds should be noted and can be treated with incision and drainage. Intra-abdominal abscess presents with abdominal pain and persistent fevers. It is confirmed with CT scan and treated by percutaneous drainage and antibiotics [6]. Attempts to prevent pneumonia include early ambulation and pulmonary toilet (incentive spirometer, deep breathing exercises). Once diagnosed, it should be treated with an appropriate course of antibiotics.

18.5   Stricture

LSG is thought of as a less technically challenging procedure than other weight loss surgeries; however, the successful creation of the long gastric tube requires considerable expertise. Stricture can occur for a number of technical reasons including the use of small bougie sizes and asymmetrical lateral traction while creating the sleeve which results in twisting. Chronic inflammation from staple line leaks can also result in stricture. Overall stricture rate is approximately 2–3.5 % [9].

Most strictures are symptomatic within the first 6 weeks following surgery and often present when the patient is progressed to solid food [5]. Occasionally they will present acutely due to tissue edema. Patients will complain of persistent reflux symptoms, often unrelated to oral intake. An upper gastrointestinal series or endoscopic evaluation is typically diagnostic [6].

Management consists of initial observation and multiple sessions of endoscopic balloon dilation. Injection of botulinum toxin into the pylorus has also been attempted [9]. If these attempts fail, surgical intervention may be necessary including seromyotomy (cutting of the stomach muscle) and conversion to a Roux-en-Y gastric bypass [6].

18.6   Nutritional Deficiencies

Nutritional deficiencies are common both before and after bariatric surgery because of impaired absorption and decreased oral intake. Nutrients most commonly affected after LSG include vitamin B12, vitamin D, folate, iron, and zinc. In general these deficits are less severe after LSG than Roux-en-Y gastric bypass. Routine blood work is warranted, and vitamin and mineral deficiencies should be corrected as necessary [6].

Review Questions

1. A patient returns to the emergency department postoperative day 7 from a laparoscopic sleeve gastrectomy. She complains of acute onset of shortness of breath and you note a heart rate of 130. She denies abdominal tenderness and her incisions are healing well. What is the most likely diagnosis for her presenting complaint?

   A. Staple line leak
   B. Pulmonary embolism
   C. Intra-abdominal abscess

D. Gastroesophageal reflux disease
E. Deep vein thrombosis

2. Which diagnostic modality would you use to confirm your diagnostic suspicion in the patient from question 1?

A. Computed tomography (CT) of the abdomen and pelvis
B. Endoscopy
C. Spiral CT angiogram (CTA) of the chest
D. Ultrasound of the legs
E. Esophageal pH monitoring

3. What is your treatment plan for the patient in question 1?

A. Diagnostic laparoscopy and placement of omental patch.
B. Heparin drip followed by long-term anticoagulation.
C. Percutaneous drainage by interventional radiology.
D. Proton pump inhibitor.
E. This complication can be controlled endoscopically.

4. Your patient is now postoperative day 1 from an LSG. She has received all of her medications including her metoprolol. She complains of left-sided abdominal pain and dizziness when standing. Her HR is 75, BP is 110/65, and RR is 16. You alert the resident of these findings, and initial laboratory assessment shows an increase in creatinine as well as a 3 g drop in hemoglobin. You suspect:

A. Normal postoperative findings
B. Dehydration
C. Beta-blocker overdose
D. Intra-abdominal hemorrhage
E. Staple line leak

5. Just before initiating a blood transfusion for the patient in question 4, you repeat her vital signs. Her blood pressure is now 75/40 and HR is 95. The best treatment is:

A. Take the patient immediately to the OR.
B. Continue with planned blood transfusion.
C. 1 L normal saline bolus.
D. Repeat hemoglobin.
E. Initiate Levophed drip.

Answers

1. The answer is *B*. When a bariatric patient presents with tachycardia and shortness of breath, your first suspicion should always be pulmonary embolism. Staple line leak and intra-abdominal abscess may also become apparent within the first week postoperatively; however, we would expect both of these to present with some combination of abdominal pain and

fevers. GERD can present with asthma-like symptoms but would classically cause epigastric burning not tachycardia. The patient may also have a DVT which leads to PE; however, leg swelling and/or erythema is not her presenting complaint.

2. The answer is *C*. The diagnostic study of choice to diagnose PE is spiral CT angiogram (CTA) of the chest. Other diagnostic options would include ventilation/perfusion scan if the patient was unable to receive contrast dye. CT of the abdomen and pelvis would be useful for diagnosis of a leak. Endoscopy would help evaluate for stricture or ulcer. Ultrasound of the legs, specifically the venous system, would be the diagnostic test for suspected DVT. Esophageal pH monitoring plays an important role in evaluation of reflux.

3. The answer is *B*. The treatment for PE is initiation of anticoagulation followed by 6 months of therapeutic anticoagulation as an outpatient. If this patient has a previous history of venous thromboembolism, they will require lifelong anticoagulation. Diagnostic laparoscopy may be useful if a leak is suspected. Intra-abdominal abscesses should be assessed by interventional radiology for drainage. Initial treatment for reflux is with the initiation of proton pump inhibitors. Endoscopic therapy can be employed for the treatment of bleeding ulcers and therapeutic dilation of strictures.

4. The answer is *D*. The most likely cause of this scenario is intra-abdominal hemorrhage. Beta-blockers will often mask the tachycardic response expected from a patient in hemorrhagic shock. Laboratory values may often lag behind; however, in this case, our suspicion is confirmed by the 3 g drop in hemoglobin.

5. The answer is *A*. This patient has now become unstable and should be taken to the OR for exploration making this the best answer. In reality she may initially require a saline bolus to improve her hypotension. The blood transfusion should also be continued. A repeat hemoglobin is not necessary, and waiting for this result before taking action could be deadly. The patient is experiencing hemorrhagic shock. The treatment is replacement of volume, not vasopressors.

References

1. Young M, Gebhart A, Phelen M et al (2015) Use and outcomes of laparoscopic sleeve gastrectomy vs laparoscopic gastric bypass: analysis of the American College of Surgeons NSQIP. J Am Coll Surg 220(5):880–885
2. Durmush E, Ermerak G, Durmush D (2014) Short-term outcomes of sleeve gastrectomy for morbid obesity: does staple line reinforcement matter. Obes Surg 24:1109–1116
3. Sakran N, Goitein D, Raziel A et al (2013) Gastric leaks after sleeve gastrectomy: a multicenter experience with 2,834 patients. Surg Endosc 27(1):240–245
4. Rached A, Basile M, Masri H (2014) Gastric leaks post sleeve gastrectomy: review of its prevention and management. World J Gastroenterol 20(38):13904–13910

5. Rosenthal R, International Sleeve Gastrectomy Expert Panel (2012) International sleeve gastrectomy expert panel consensus statement. Surg Obes Relat Dis 8:8–19

6. Sarkhosh K, Birch D, Sharma A, Karmali S (2013) Complications associated with laparoscopic sleeve gastrectomy for morbid obesity: a surgeon's guide. Can J Surg 56(5):347–352

7. Finks J, English W, Carlin A et al (2012) Predicting risk for venous thromboembolism with bariatric surgery. Ann Surg 255(6):1100–1104

8. Spaniolas K, Kasten K, Sippey M et al (2016) Pulmonary embolism and gastrointestinal leak following bariatric surgery: when do major complications occur. Surg Obes Relat Dis 12(2):379–383

9. Vilallonga R, Himpens J, Vrande S (2013) Laparoscopic management of persistent strictures after laparoscopic sleeve gastrectomy. Obes Surg 23:1655–1661

General Overview of the Laparoscopic Roux-en-Y Gastric Bypass

19

Roshin Thomas

The laparoscopic Roux-en-Y gastric bypass (LRYGB) is both a restrictive and malabsorptive procedure. Patients are placed under general anesthesia for the procedure. During the procedure, the stomach is made into a very small pouch. This is the restrictive part of the procedure by reducing the amount of food that can be consumed during meals. Once the stomach is stapled into a small pouch, the antrum, pylorus, duodenum, and 40 cm of the jejunum are divided. The jejunum at this point is attached to the stomach. The bypassed duodenum is then attached to the jejunum 80–150 cm from its site of attachment to the stomach. This is where Roux-en-Y gastric bypass got its name [1]. This is the malabsorptive part of the procedure.

In comparison to the gastric sleeve, patients lose weight faster with a bypass. They lose about 60–80 % of their weight within the first year, whereas with a sleeve, the weight loss is slower within the first year. However, unlike a sleeve, gastric bypasses have the potential risk of dumping syndrome.

Dumping syndrome occurs when a large bolus of food enters the stomach and small intestine too rapidly. It can be divided into both early and late stages. The early stage occurs within 15–30 min after eating. The late stage occurs hours after a meal. In the early stage, the large fluid bolus causes hyperosmolar shifts in the small intestines. This in turn draws large amounts of fluids into the gut lumen and causes overdistention. This leads to symptoms such as nausea, vomiting, bloating, diarrhea, and fatigue. The symptoms of the late stage of dumping occur due to hypoglycemia. In reaction to the large hyperosmotic load and fluid shifts, the pancreas releases a large amount of insulin into the bloodstream. These symptoms include diaphoresis, weakness, and fatigue. The simple solution to this is to eat smaller portions [1].

Like any surgery, the common complications of the bypass include bleeding. With morbid obesity comes other comorbid conditions such as diabetes, coronary

R. Thomas, DO
Department of General Surgery, Rowan University, Stratford, NJ, USA
e-mail: thomasrm@rowan.edu

© Springer International Publishing Switzerland 2017
A. Loveitt et al. (eds.), *Passing the Certified Bariatric Nurses Exam*,
DOI 10.1007/978-3-319-41703-5_19

85

artery disease, and hypertension. These conditions place the patients at higher risk for infections, both intra-abdominal and wound, MIs, and DVT/PE.

During the immediate postoperative course, important cues to be aware of are tachycardia, tachypnea, fever, low urine output, and low blood pressure. Other complications are nausea, vomiting, swelling in lower extremities, and leukocytosis. An elevated heart rate may represent a fever, dehydration, leak, pain, anxiety, or even a pulmonary embolism (PE). Causes for low urine output include dehydration, bleeding, or sometimes urinary retention as a complication of anesthesia. Shortness of breath could be secondary to pain. However, you must rule out a PE or cardiac event.

Long-term complications related to the LRYGB may include malnutrition and vitamin deficiencies. The most common of these deficiencies are calcium, iron, and B_{12}. As mentioned before, gastric dumping may occur. Other complications are dehydration, strictures at the anastomotic sites, internal hernias leading to small bowel obstructions, fistulas between the pouch and the remnant stomach, bleeding, and cholelithiasis. Patients may develop ulcers at the anastomotic sites, called marginal ulcers, especially if they continue to smoke [2].

Patients are expected to stay in the hospital for an average of 2–3 days after the surgery. Most patients get an upper GI series on postoperative day 1 to rule out a leak or obstruction. Once they have a negative upper GI, they are started on a bariatric stage 1 diet. They are encouraged to take in at least 64 oz of fluid daily.

General follow-up is a week to 2 weeks after the surgery. Following the initial visit, they are followed up after 3 months. During this visit, a BMP and CBC are checked. At the sixth-month follow-up, liver function tests, protein and albumin, iron, total iron-binding capacity, ferritin, vitamin B_{12}, folic acid, calcium, and parathyroid hormone are checked. The patients are then asked to follow up once a year after that, and the same labs are checked and evaluated at each visit. Pregnancy is contraindicated for at least 18 months after surgery because of the rapid weight loss and nutritional requirements [3].

References

1. Mullholand MW et al (2012) Greenfield's surgery: scientific principles & practice, 5th edn. LWW, Philadelphia
2. Ellsmere J. (2016) Late Complications of bariatric surgical operations. UpToDate.
3. Oregon Health & Science University (2016) Post-op instructions. OHSU Bariatric Services. [Online].

Laparoscopic Roux-en-Y Gastric Bypass: The Procedure

20

Roshin Thomas

The concept of the laparoscopic Roux-en-Y gastric bypass (LRYGB) is both restriction and malabsorption (mostly fat malabsorption since most of the duodenum is bypassed). This procedure was initially described in the 1960s by Drs. Mason and Ito [1]. Prior to being a weight loss tool, this procedure was performed for patients with chronic ulcers. However, the long-term weight loss noted in these patients led to the conclusion that it could also be used to help patients with morbid obesity. Over the course of the years since it has been introduced, this procedure has undergone multiple modifications to become the procedure that it is now.

The procedure involves four major steps, the order of which may vary by surgeon:

1. Creation of a 15-mL stapled gastric pouch
2. Gastrojejunostomy – connection between the gastric pouch and jejunum which creates the Roux limb
3. 75- to 150-cm Roux limb
4. Jejunojejunostomy – connection between the two limbs of jejunum which creates the bypass

20.1 Patient Positioning, Access, and Port Placement

After informed consent is obtained, the patient is placed supine on the operating room table. These tables are designed to hold someone who weighs up to 800 lbs; secure straps are placed across the patient above and below the waist. The patient's arms are extended and placed on padded arm boards. This is to prevent tension on

R. Thomas, DO
Department of General Surgery, Rowan University, Stratford, NJ, USA
e-mail: thomasrm@rowan.edu

© Springer International Publishing Switzerland 2017
A. Loveitt et al. (eds.), *Passing the Certified Bariatric Nurses Exam*,
DOI 10.1007/978-3-319-41703-5_20

Fig. 20.1 Roux-en-Y
gastric bypass

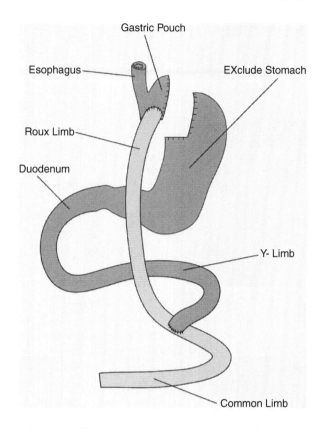

the shoulders and the brachial plexus [1]. After general anesthesia is induced, the patient's abdomen is prepped widely.

The surgeon generally stands on the right with the assistants on the opposite side, facing the surgeon. Placement of port sites varies with surgeons, but most bariatric procedures require five to six port sites [2]. A liver retractor is placed through one of the ports to help expose the stomach.

20.2   Creation of the Gastric Pouch

The LRYGB can begin with the creation of the gastric pouch (Fig. 20.1). A tunnel is created beneath the upper portion of the stomach, being careful to avoid injury to the diaphragm, spleen, and esophagus. An endoscopic stapler is then used to divide the stomach, first horizontally and then vertically to create a gastric pouch of about 10–15 mL [1].

20.3   Creation of the Biliary Pancreatic Limb

The most proximal portion of the small bowel is located and then measured approximately 50 cm distally where the jejunum is transected using an endoscopic stapler.

20.4   Creation of Gastrojejunostomy

A connection between the stomach and the previously transected jejunum is made to create the Roux limb which will carry gastric contents from the newly created gastric pouch directly to the distal jejunum creating the bypass. There are many ways to create this connection using a variety of stapling devices or by laparoscopic suturing [2].

20.5   Creation of Jejunojejunostomy

The jejunojejunostomy (JJ) is the connection between the Roux limb (which carries the pouch contents) and the biliopancreatic limb (which carries the remnant stomach contents). The point where this connection is made marks the end of the bypass. Prior to creating the jejunojejunostomy, the surgeon measures out between 75 and 150 cm of the jejunum. This is then determined to be the area where the JJ anastomosis will be created. The pieces of bowel are connected using staplers or sewing techniques similar to those used for the gastrojejunostomy.

There are several holes in the mesentery of the bowel which are created when making these connections. It is important to close these as it may be a potential site for bowel to slip through in the future, called an internal hernia. This can have devastating consequences including death of nearly all the small bowel.

The last step many surgeons perform is a leak test. The abdomen is filled with fluid and the gastrojejunostomy is submerged. An endoscope is placed in the stomach, and air is inflated to examine for occult leaks. If a leak is noted, it is repaired.

Once it is confirmed that there is no leak, the abdomen is inspected for any signs of bleeding, and the bowel is laid in appropriate anatomic position, the ports are removed, the pneumoperitoneum is released, and incisions are closed.

Review Questions

1. Which of the following is not a part of the RYGBP?

   A. Creation of a jejunojejunostomy
   B. Small gastric pouch
   C. Connecting the biliopancreatic limb to the stomach
   D. Creation of gastrojejunostomy

2. Why is it imperative to close defects in the mesentery where bowel connections are made?

   A. Prevent future internal hernias.
   B. It helps secure the gastrojejunal anastomotic site.
   C. This stops small vessel bleeding caused during dissection of the omentum.
   D. Prevents abscess formation.

3. The following are options for creation of gastrojejunal anastomosis EXCEPT:

   A. Using an energy device
   B. Using the Endo GIA stapler
   C. Using an anvil-stapling device
   D. Laparoscopically sewing the anastomosis

4. What is the starting point used to measure the jejunum?

   A. Gastrocolic ligament
   B. Phrenoesophageal ligament
   C. Ligament of Treitz
   D. Hepatoduodenal ligament

Answers

1. The answer is *C*. The biliopancreatic limb is the section of the small bowel which includes the duodenum and very proximal jejunum. It functions to drain the remnant stomach, biliary system, and pancreas which produce the digestive juices. These digestive juices then rejoin the Roux limb at the jejunojenunostomy after food has already traveled through much of the intestine, creating the malabsorptive portion of the LRYGB. If the biliopancreatic limb were connected back to the stomach, it would create a loop!

2. The answer is *A*. One of the most feared complications of the LRYGB is an internal hernia. When portions of the small bowel slip through mesenteric defects, the blood supply can become compromised and the bowel can die. For this reason, these defects are typically closed.

3. The answer is *A*. Remember, an anastomosis is the connection between two pieces of intestine. It is created using a stapling or suturing device. Using an energy device would result in cutting, not connecting the tissue.

4. The answer is *C*. This is surely beyond the level of knowledge required for the CBN exam, but the ligament of Treitz is an important landmark for surgeons. It marks the transition from the duodenum to jejunum and is typically the most proximal portion of the small bowel encountered in the LRYGB. It has important embryological and anatomical implications.

References

1. Schauer P (2003) Laparoscopic gastric bypass surgery: current technique. J Laparoendosc Adv Surg Tech A 13(4):229–239
2. Zeni T (2009) Laparoscopic Roux-en-Y gastric bypass. In: Atlas of minimally invasive surgery. Elsevier, Philadelphia. pp 75–77

Roux-en-Y Gastric Bypass: Pros and Cons

21

Roshin Thomas

With the abundance of informational material freely available to patients, they often present to the surgeon with a preconceived idea of which weight loss procedure is right for them. It is up to their surgeon and their team, however, to help the patient weigh the pros and cons of each procedure and make a final determination.

21.1 Pros of the Laparoscopic Roux-en-Y Gastric Bypass

- Potentially higher excess weight loss
- More effective control of diabetes
- Better control of cravings
- Better control of reflux/Barrett's esophagus

21.2 Cons

- Requires permanent changes to the anatomy.
- Multiple anastomoses which can form strictures or ulcers.
- Potential for internal hernias.
- Lifetime vitamin supplementation is required.

While all the procedures enable speedy weight loss, it is studied and concluded that after 1 year, the LRYGB has a higher percentage of excess weight loss when compared to laparoscopic sleeve gastrectomy (LSG), 84.2 % vs. 66.1 %. At the 5-year mark, patients were able to maintain 65–70 % of excess weight loss [1]. LRYGB is effective for patients with a higher BMI due to the higher percentage of

R. Thomas, DO
Department of General Surgery, Rowan University, Stratford, NJ, USA
e-mail: thomasrm@rowan.edu

© Springer International Publishing Switzerland 2017
A. Loveitt et al. (eds.), *Passing the Certified Bariatric Nurses Exam*,
DOI 10.1007/978-3-319-41703-5_21

weight loss. Meta-analysis also demonstrates that LRYGB is more effective than LSG for the treatment of type 2 diabetes mellitus and metabolic syndrome [2]. Studies have shown that 90% of patients see an improvement in their DM and high blood pressure. Patients also note that their sleep apnea no longer poses a problem, and their use of CPAP had significantly reduced [1]. There were also significant improvements in their gastric reflux and osteoarthritis. The LRYGB is also more effective for people who crave foods that are high in sugar or fat. This is directly related to dumping syndrome that occurs when such foods are consumed. This then discourages patients from eating unhealthy [3].

Although the abovementioned facts make the LRYGB appealing to many patients, the complications or disadvantages of this procedure are more severe in nature as well. Unlike gastric banding, this procedure results in permanent disruption of the anatomy. Once a patient undergoes a LRYGB, it is rarely reversed. The procedure itself is more technically challenging, which leads to longer operative time as well as longer hospital course [3]. Studies have also shown that the rates of readmission were higher in LRYGB compared to LSG. It was also noted that the initial length of stay in the hospital immediately post-op had a correlation to the readmission rate as well [4].

With multiple areas of anastomoses, the chance of a leak is increased. The anastomotic areas are also at risk for developing marginal ulcers, particularly at the jejunal side. Patients also develop strictures at their sites of anastomoses. When compared to the other weight loss procedures, LRYGB has a higher risk of internal hernias – three areas in particular are potential sites. Due to the malabsorptive nature of the procedure, patients are also at a higher risk of nutritional deficiencies such as deficit in iron, vitamin B12, iron, calcium, and folate [3]. Patients will require lifelong supplementation of vitamin and minerals as well as long-term follow-up with their surgeon and dietitian. When compared to gastric banding or sleeve gastrectomy, patients that undergo a LRYGB may experience dumping syndrome which is described in detail elsewhere.

Review Questions

1. Which of the following procedures does *NOT* result in permanent distortion of the patient's anatomy?

   A. The laparoscopic Roux-en-Y gastric bypass
   B. The laparoscopic adjustable band
   C. The laparoscopic sleeve gastrectomy
   D. The duodenal switch

2. A patient with a BMI of 35 presents inquiring about weight loss surgery. He has multiple friends who have had great success with their laparoscopic sleeve gastrectomies. You notice that his past medical history includes type 2 diabetes and Barrett's esophagus. You recommend:

   A. The patient proceeds with sleeve gastrectomy, it worked for his friends, and they will be a good support group.
   B. The patient should consider an adjustable band. His weight loss is likely to be similar to that of his friends, and he can always have the band removed.

    C. The duodenal switch would be his best option because it will lead to more weight loss.

    D. The patient should consider a gastric bypass; it will lead to better control of his diabetes and limit further reflux.

3. Which of the following is considered a marginal ulcer?

    A. An ulcer occurring at the anastomosis between the stomach and jejunum

    B. An ulcer occurring at the gastroesophageal junction

    C. An ulcer occurring in the gastric remnant

    D. An ulcer occurring within the biliopancreatic limb

4. You are interviewing a patient 1 year after LRYGB, and he is happy with the results. He has lost 50 % of his excess body weight and is off of his diabetes and hypertension medications. He inquires how long he will need to take his multivitamin as he would like to be completely "pill-free." You answer:

    A. You should follow up with your medical doctor immediately; your HgA1C is probably through the roof!

    B. The cardiologist will surely be unhappy that you stopped your antihypertensives.

    C. You will never be "pill-free" because you will need to take your multivitamin lifelong.

    D. You're a year out from surgery and doing great; don't worry about that pesky pill!

Answers

1. The answer is *B*. The laparoscopic adjustable band is placed by creating a window around the fundus of the stomach; however, there is no cutting of the GI tract itself. The LRYGB, while technically reversible, does require cutting and re-routing portions of the GI tract and results in permanent changes. The sleeve gastrectomy and duodenal switch involve cutting and removing a portion of the stomach and cannot be reversed.

2. The answer is *D*. The LRYGB has been shown to be superior in controlling diabetes and is also indicated when a patient has severe reflux and/or Barrett's esophagus. A sleeve gastrectomy would be a poor choice in this patient as it is contraindicated with Barrett's. The adjustable band has *inferior* weight loss when compared to the LRYGB. A duodenal switch may indeed lead to superior weight loss but in this patient with a BMI of only 35 may be too drastic of a procedure.

3. The answer is *A*. A marginal ulcer is a unique complication to the Roux-en-Y bypass and occurs at the gastrojejunal anastomosis, typically on the jejunal side. Smoking and the use of NSAIDs are common risk factors, and these should be avoided. Patients present with abdominal pain, nausea, and vomiting (sometimes bloody). They are typically diagnosed by endoscopy and treated with PPIs.

4. The answer is *C*. Many patients have a remarkable (and often immediate) control of blood sugar and hypertension after LRYGB, and with this patient's weight loss, he likely does not need to take these medications any longer. He should, however, continue taking a multivitamin for the rest of his life as the malabsorption created by the LRYGB can lead to vitamin deficiencies despite well-rounded diets.

References

1. Skinner A, Yosuke M (2012) Sleeve gastrectomy versus Roux-en-Y gastric bypass: a retrospective review of weight-loss and resolution of co-morbidities–SAGES abstract archives. SAGES. [Online]
2. Li JF, Lai D, Ni B, Sun KX (2013) Comparison of laparoscopic Roux-en-Y Gastric bypass with laparoscopic sleeve gastrectomy for morbid obesity or type 2 diabetes mellitus: a meta-analysis of randomized controlled trials. Can J Surg 56(6):E158–64
3. ASMBS (2015) Bariatric surgery procedures. American Society for Metabolic and Bariatric Surgery. [Online]. Available: https://asmbs.org/patients/bariatric-surgery-procedures. [Accessed Apr 2016]
4. MBSAQIP (2014) 2014 Metabolic and Bariatric Surgery Accreditation and Quality Improvement Program (MBSAQIP),Qualified Clinical Data Registry (QCDR) Non-PQRS Measures Specifications. [Online]. Available: https://www.facs.org/quality-programs/mbsaqip. Accessed Apr 2016.

Roux-en-Y Gastric Bypass: Recognizing and Treating Complications

22

Roshin Thomas

Postoperative complications following laparoscopic Roux-en-Y gastric bypass (LRYGB) can be broadly grouped into early and late complications. Complications that occur within the 2-week postoperative period are considered an early complication. Complications after the second postoperative week are considered late complications.

Like any surgery, the common complications of the bypass include bleeding and infection. With morbid obesity comes other comorbid conditions such as diabetes, coronary artery disease, and hypertension. These conditions place the patients at higher risk for infections – both intra-abdominal and wound, myocardial infarctions, and DVT/PE. Important cues to be aware of are tachycardia, tachypnea, fever, low urine output, and low blood pressure. Additionally, nausea, vomiting, swelling in lower extremities, and leukocytosis may point to larger underlying issues.

22.1 Early Complications

22.1.1 Anastomotic Leaks

One of the most dreaded and quite possibly devastating complications of this procedure, with a mortality rate of nearly 50 %, is an anastomotic leak. A multivariate study of 3000 patients who underwent LRYGB concluded that an anastomotic leak was one of the strongest independent risk factors for postoperative death. The incidence of leak is relatively low at 0.4–5.2 % [1].

The most common site for a leak is at the gastrojejunal anastomosis. Generally, clinical signs such as tachycardia, fevers, nausea/vomiting, and abdominal pain are indicators of a leak. A recent study concluded that sustained tachycardia with a

R. Thomas, DO
Department of General Surgery, Rowan University, Stratford, NJ, USA
e-mail: thomasrm@rowan.edu

© Springer International Publishing Switzerland 2017
A. Loveitt et al. (eds.), *Passing the Certified Bariatric Nurses Exam*,
DOI 10.1007/978-3-319-41703-5_22

heart rate in excess of 120 beats per minute was a good indicator [2]. Early operative management is typically the treatment for leaks following LRYGB. The goal of the operation is to find and repair the leak, remove gastric contents from the abdomen, and place drains [1]. Patients are then treated with IV antibiotics and fluids. They are also maintained NPO until their symptoms improve.

22.1.2 Postoperative Bleeding

There are two types of postoperative hemorrhage that can occur. The first is intra-abdominal where the bleeding occurs along the staple lines, at the anastomoses, or the gastric pouch. The second site of bleeding can occur *within* the bowel at the previously mentioned sites. Once again clinical signs and laboratory results may be the initial indicators of a bleed. Tachycardia, drop in the hemoglobin level and/or urine output, and excessive bloody output from the drain or the incisions are a few such signs and symptoms. Surgical intervention is prudent at this point. The source of the bleed is identified and controlled, and the abdominal cavity is evacuated of any clots that may have developed.

22.1.3 Dumping Syndrome

As mentioned earlier, dumping syndrome occurs when a large bolus of food enters the stomach and small intestines too rapidly. It can be divided into both early and late stages. The early stage occurs within 15–30 min after eating. The late stage occurs hours after a meal. In the early stage, the large fluid bolus causes hyperosmolar shifts in the small intestines. This is in turn draws large amounts of fluids into the gut lumen and causes overdistention. This causes symptoms such as nausea, vomiting, bloating, diarrhea, and fatigue. The symptoms of the late stage of dumping occur due to hypoglycemia. In reaction to the large hyperosmotic load and fluid shifts, the pancreas releases a large amount of insulin into the bloodstream. These symptoms include diaphoresis, weakness, and fatigue. The simple solution to this is to eat smaller portions [3].

22.1.4 DVT

Deep vein thrombosis (DVT) with resultant pulmonary embolism is the most common cause of death after bariatric surgery. Although the incidence of such an event is only 2 %, the mortality associated with it is around 20–30 % [4]. In order to avoid such a complication, patients are given chemoprophylaxis in the form of subcutaneous heparin or Lovenox. Perhaps the most important intervention is to encourage early ambulation including postoperative day 0. Sequential compression devices are applied to allow constant circulation of blood in the lower extremities.

22.2   Late Complications

22.2.1 Marginal Ulceration

This is an ulcer that develops at or near the gastrojejunal anastomotic line. Most patients complain of burning epigastric pain. Factors that contribute to ulcer formation are NSAIDs, smoking, and *H. pylori*. These ulcers can be treated with proton pump inhibitors (PPIs), sucralfate, and conservative therapy. However, in complicated marginal ulcer (perforation or bleeding), the solution is surgical. Once again the goals of surgery are to identify the bleed or locate the ulcer, control bleeding, and repair the site of perforation.

22.2.2 Small Bowel Obstruction

The most common cause of small bowel obstructions after a LRYGB is an internal hernia. An internal hernia is defined as herniation of bowel through a mesenteric defect. In the process of dividing bowel and mesentery to create two new anastomoses, we are creating three potential sites for internal hernias. Patients present with colicky abdominal pain, nausea, and vomiting. This can be episodic or continuous in nature. Some may complain of abdominal distention. CT scan with oral and IV contrast may sometimes be helpful in diagnosing this condition. Once recognized, patients are maintained NPO, adequately resuscitated with IV fluids, and then taken to the operating room. An additional cause of small bowel obstruction may be adhesions that are formed postoperatively [1].

22.2.3 Strictures/Stenosis

Strictures can occur as a long-term complication of the LRYGB. Patients may present in weeks to months with progressive dysphagia and inability to tolerate food. They may also complain of daily vomiting with little or no abdominal pain. Increased tension around the anastomotic region and ischemia are the two main causes for strictures. A diagnostic upper GI with contrast is initially performed to note the anatomy as well as the movement of contrast. Endoscopic dilation is successful in most patients. However, if this approach does not work, once again surgical intervention will be necessary. In this case, the strictured area is resected, and a new anastomosis is created [1].

22.2.4 Nutritional Deficiencies

Due to reconfiguration of the GI system and poor oral intake, patients may experience some nutritional deficiencies. The duodenum is the site of absorption of iron and folate. The stomach produces intrinsic factor which is a cofactor that is needed to absorb B12 from the gut. When a large part of the stomach is bypassed, patients also experience B12 deficiencies. Patients are referred to a dietician as well as given iron and folate supplements. Routine blood work may also be necessary to detect and monitor mineral and vitamin deficiencies [5].

Review Questions

1. Which of the following is not a common early complication after bypass surgery?

   A. Ileus
   B. DVT
   C. Bleeding
   D. Strictures
   E. Dumping syndrome

2. In dumping syndrome the early symptoms are caused due to?

   A. Hypoglycemia
   B. Hyperosmolar shifts
   C. Late ambulation
   D. Dehydration
   E. Pain

3. All of the following are causes of marginal ulcers *except*:

   A. NSAIDs
   B. Cigarette smoking
   C. *H. pylori*
   D. Alcohol abuse

4. The following are signs of a bleeding patient *except*:

   A. Tachycardia
   B. Bloody drain output
   C. Drop in urine output
   D. Drop in hemoglobin
   E. Bilateral lower extremity swelling

Answers

1. The answer is *D*. While it is possible for the surgeon to create a mechanical stricture during the procedure, most strictures typically present after the patient leaves the hospital. Often when their diet is advanced and they are considered a late complication.
2. The answer is *B*. Dumping syndrome occurs in early and late stages. The early stage occurs after a food bolus enters the GI symptom leading to rapid shifts of fluids into the bowel and occurs within minutes of eating. The late stage is due to hypoglycemia caused by overproduction of insulin in response to these shifts.

3. The answer is *D*. NSAIDs, smoking, and *H. pylori* are all implicated in the production of marginal ulcers. Alcohol is also not encouraged, but this is because the rapid absorption makes the patient's response unpredictable. It has not been shown to lead to ulcers.

4. The answer is *E*. Bilateral lower extremity swelling is more commonly associated with DVT or fluid overload, only rarely would it be associated with bleeding.

References

1. Griffith PS, Birch DW, Sharma AM, Karmali S (2012) Managing complications associated with laparoscopic Roux-en-Y gastric bypass for morbid obesity. Can J Surg 55(5):329–336
2. Bellorin O, Abdemur A, Sucandy I, Szomstein S, Rosenthal RJ (2011) Understanding the significance, reasons and patterns of abnormal vital signs after gastric bypass for morbid obesity. Obes Surg 21(6):707–713
3. Carvajal SH, Mulvihill SJ (1994) Postgastrectomy syndromes: dumping and diarrhea. Gastroenterol Clin North Am 23:261–279
4. Byrne TK (2001) Complications of surgery for obesity. Surg Clin North Am 81:1181–1193
5. Schauer PR (2003) Laparoscopic gastric bypass surgery: current technique. J Laparoendosc Adv Surg Tech A 13(4):229–239, Reuters

Biliopancreatic Diversion with Duodenal Switch (BPD/DS)

23

Marc A. Neff

The biliopancreatic diversion with duodenal switch – abbreviated as BPD/DS – is a two-part procedure. Scopinaro first performed the biliopancreatic diversion (BPD) which was designed to be a safe malabsorptive procedure [1]. The first part of the procedure is very similar to the sleeve gastrectomy and was actually where the sleeve gastrectomy first originated. In the second part, roughly ¾ of the small intestine is bypassed (Fig. 23.1).

Malabsorption of calories and nutrients occurs via two mechanisms. First, the bile and pancreatic fluids and other digestive enzymes eventually join the ingested food – but at a point in the distal small intestine (ileum) where there is much less chance for complete breakdown and absorption, approximately 50–100 cm from the colon. The undigested fat consumed by the patient can cause gas and loose, foul-smelling bowel movements. The second mechanism through which malabsorption occurs is by decreasing the amount of small intestine through which the ingested food passes. With so little of the intestine with which food is in contact, less nutrients can be absorbed [1].

Patients also experience changes in gut hormones in a manner that impacts hunger and satiety as well as blood sugar control. The BPD/DS is considered by many to be the most effective surgery for the treatment of diabetes and to have the greatest total amount and greatest sustained long-term weight loss [1].

The BPD/DS can be performed laparoscopically, but this operation is more demanding technically than the Roux-en-Y gastric bypass and should only be performed by fellowship-trained surgeons in experienced centers.

M.A. Neff, MD, FACS, FASMBS
General Surgery, Kennedy Health Alliance, Cherry Hill, NJ, USA
e-mail: M.Neff@kennedyhealth.org

© Springer International Publishing Switzerland 2017
A. Loveitt et al. (eds.), *Passing the Certified Bariatric Nurses Exam*,
DOI 10.1007/978-3-319-41703-5_23

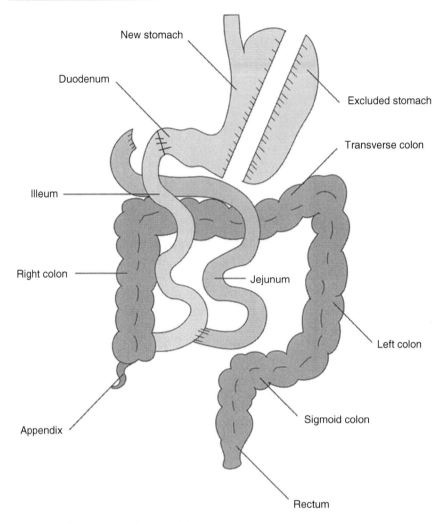

Fig. 23.1 Biliopancreatic diversion with duodenal switch

23.1 Advantages

1. Results in the greatest total and sustained weight loss of the commonly performed bariatric procedures, i.e., 70–80 % excess weight loss or greater, at 5 year follow-up
2. Allows patients to eventually eat near "normal" meals with increased amount of food intake compared to the bypass and band with less food intolerance
3. Reduces the absorption of fat by more than 70 %
4. Causes favorable changes in gut hormones to reduce appetite and improve satiety

5. Is the most effective against diabetes
6. More rapid weight loss compared with other weight loss surgeries

23.2   Disadvantages

1. Has the highest complication rates compared to all other weight loss surgeries.
2. Has a greater potential to cause protein deficiencies and long-term vitamin and minerals deficiencies.
3. Compliance with follow-up dietician visits and strict adherence to dietary and vitamin supplementation guidelines are critical.
4. Diarrhea and foul-smelling gas, with an average of 3–4 loose bowel movements a day.
5. Malabsorption of fat-soluble vitamins (vitamins A, D, E, and K).

Conclusions

The BPD/DS is a safe alternative to the old-fashioned jejunal-ileal bypass. There is very good initial and sustained weight loss. The major mechanism at work is malabsorption. The procedure is best performed at centers that have adequate technical expertise to perform such a complicated and higher-risk surgical procedure and at centers capable of providing the appropriate dietary counseling and follow-up necessary to prevent the associated nutritional deficiencies. Follow-up for this procedure, given the degree of malabsorption, really should be considered mandatory and lifelong.

Review Questions

1. The main mechanism for weight loss in the BPD/DS is:

   A. Through restriction
   B. Through malabsorption
   C. Through changes in gut hormones
   D. Because of steatorrhea

2. Compared to the gastric band and sleeve gastrectomy, patients who undergo a BPD/DS experience:

   A. Faster weight loss
   B. Greater sustained weight loss
   C. More risk for nutritional deficiencies
   D. All of the above

3. Which of the following nutritional deficiencies is not typically seen after a BPD/DS?

   A. Malabsorption of fat-soluble vitamins D, E, and K
   B. Vitamin A deficiency, which causes night blindness
   C. Folate deficiency

D. Iron deficiency
E. Protein-calorie malnutrition

Answers

1. The answer is *B*. While all are true regarding the BPD/DS, the major mechanism of weight loss is through malabsorption of protein and fat, calories, and nutrients. Strict dietary compliance and follow-up are necessary to avoid serious nutritional deficiencies. Steatorrhea is a well-recognized phenomenon of the fat malabsorption associated with the procedure but is not specifically a mechanism for the experienced weight loss.
2. The answer is *D*. The BPD/DS is the most malabsorptive procedure currently performed by weight loss surgeons. Long-term data suggest faster weight loss and greater sustained weight loss compared with patients who have banding and sleeve gastrectomy procedures. The data even is better than traditional gastric bypass patients. These benefits are offset by a higher complication rate, higher mortality rate, and higher risk of nutritional deficiencies, both in the short and long term.
3. The answer is *C*. Fat-soluble vitamin deficiencies are well recognized after the BPD/DS. These include vitamin A deficiency which is associated with night blindness and vitamin D deficiency which is associated with osteoporosis. Iron deficiency at similar rates to that seen in the gastric bypass procedure is also common. Folate deficiency can be seen in weight loss surgery patients but is not specifically associated with the BPD/DS.

Reference

1. ASMBS (2016) Bariatric surgery procedures: biliopancreatic diversion with duodenal switch. American Society for Metabolic and Bariatric Surgery. [Online]. Available: http://asmbs.org/patients/bariatric-surgery-procedures#bpd

Special Equipment for the Bariatric Patient

Lisa Harasymczuk

The bariatric patient represents a patient population that requires dedicated hospital equipment. The standard hospital equipment is not sufficient for these patients. Hospital beds, patient chairs, OR tables, wheelchairs, radiologic tables, surgical instruments, etc., are rated for a specific weight maximum. For the bariatric patient, this needs to be taken into consideration.

When a hospital becomes accredited by the American College of Surgeons, they must meet certain standards of care for this patient population. Weight capacities must be documented by the manufacturer's specifications, and this information must be readily available to relevant staff. The staff must also be trained on this equipment and its proper usage. Centers do not need to change all of the equipment, furniture, and instruments throughout the entire facility. This requirement only applies to those areas where patients undergoing metabolic and bariatric surgery receive care, including the operating room, emergency department, radiology suite, designated metabolic and bariatric unit, and waiting areas [1]. Most equipment defined as bariatric has a 300–900 pound weight limit – though there is not a specific width or designated weight limit that defines bariatric products [2].

Entrances and routes of the bariatric patient must provide adequate space to accommodate the bariatric wheelchair (39–49 in) with a 6-foot turning radius. The typical hospital elevators will accommodate 2000–3000 pounds, which may be exceeded when considering the weight of the patient, the patient's bed, the transport staff, and other specialized equipment. The Bariatric Room Advisory Board states that the patient rooms should be 14 ft x 15 ft to sufficiently accommodate the patient and the equipment. Patient bathrooms must have floor-mounted toilets and sinks as opposed to the typical wall mount design. This allows for a higher static load. The toilets and showers must also have enough space on either

L. Harasymczuk, DO
Department of General Surgery, Rowan University, Stratford, NJ, USA
e-mail: harasymczuk@rowan.edu

© Springer International Publishing Switzerland 2017
A. Lovcitt ct al. (cds.), *Passing the Certified Bariatric Nurses Exam*,
DOI 10.1007/978-3-319-41703-5_24

side for staff assistants. All of these things must be taken into consideration when designing a bariatric unit [3].

Bariatric equipment must combine load limit, appropriate dimensions, and a design aesthetic that blends with the environment by which a patient's and caregiver's comfort and safety are ensured. A safe *working load* or working load limit is a rating for bariatric beds, lifts, and other equipment. It is the largest load that equipment can safely lift, whereas the *static load* is the maximum amount of non-moving weight a piece of equipment can bear. This would be applied to furniture, handrails, grab bars, and toilets, for example. The *dynamic load* accommodates the weight of a patient in falling motion. Dynamic load must always exceed the static load. This load rating is critical as unstable patients often will reach out to grab or lean upon items like grab bars, furniture, or railings to stop a fall. As a rule of thumb, a falling human is double their weight. If accommodating for a bariatric population of up to 900 pounds, this equipment has to withstand an impact weight – or dynamic load – of 1800 pounds. The *functional* load is the level of loading intended to be typical of hard use [3].

Another major consideration is the operating room itself. The table must be rated for 1000 pounds and have powered movement for easy patient transfer. When the bariatric patient is on the operating room table, they have a much higher risk of developing rhabdomyolysis (the breakdown of skeletal muscle due to prolonged pressure) secondary to their increased BMI and body positioning. No studies have been done to specifically detail preventative techniques, but clinically, these patients have a lower risk of developing rhabdomyolysis if they are positioned with appropriate padding on the OR table and care is taken to ensure there are no points of increased pressure. Patients have a higher risk if placed in lithotomy or lateral decubitus position, if the operation is longer than 4 h, or if the patient's BMI is greater than 50 g/m^2 [4]. The concern of developing rhabdomyolysis is the subsequent renal failure that can result. These patients need postoperative fluid resuscitation and close monitoring of their creatinine and creatinine kinase (CK) levels. Bariatric patients have died from renal failure secondary to rhabdomyolysis. Postoperative labs, skin exam, and reported muscle pain must be taken seriously in this patient population.

It is clear there are innumerous small details that add up to create a successful bariatric unit. Some additional considerations include high-capacity (weight and girth) CT scanners, hanging overhead trapeze to assist in immediate postop mobility, special equipment (AccuVein), and skilled phlebotomists to limit needle sticks. Comfort should also be considered. Many patients find their own CPAP (continuous positive airway pressure) machine and clothes to fit more comfortably than hospital-provided materials and should be encouraged to bring their own on the date of surgery.

Review Questions

1. A 24-year-old male with a BMI of 55 g/m^2 presents following outpatient workup for his laparoscopic sleeve gastrectomy. Postoperative day zero, the patient is complaining of muscle pain in his right gluteal muscle. What is the next step given this presentation?

    A. Initiating physical therapy/occupational therapy

    B. Encouraging incentive spirometry

    C. Ensuring the patient is wearing sequential compression devices

    D. Checking postoperative basic metabolic panel/creatinine kinase

2. A patient is considering bariatric surgery at your facility. They are concerned that when they were hospitalized last year, the chair in their room was not large enough for them to use comfortably. They also had difficulty during transportation to have an X-ray performed, as the wheelchair was too small. You know that your facility is a bariatric center and that all of the bariatric equipment is rated for:

    A. 0–200 pounds

    B. 200–300 pounds

    C. 300–900 pounds

    D. 200–500 pounds

3. Which of these is an important safety consideration in the bathroom of bariatric patients?

    A. Floor-mounted toilets.

    B. Tile flooring.

    C. Large bath tub.

    D. Removable shower head.

4. Postoperatively, the only bed available for a patient who underwent a laparoscopic Roux-en-Y gastric bypass with a BMI of 45 g/m^2 is a standard inpatient bed. This bed will be sufficient for the patient, as they do not require a specialty bed.

    A. True

    B. False

5. A 42-year-old male is postoperative day one from a laparoscopic sleeve gastrectomy. His morning lab values are below. What physical exam finding would best correlate with your suspicion given these values?

Na 135, K 4.5, BUN 40, Cr 1.9, CK 5000, Hgb 12.5, Hct 35, WBC 11.2, Plt 230

    A. Pale mucous membranes

    B. Tachypnea

    C. Exquisite tenderness to palpation of the left thigh

    D. Coarse breath sounds

Answers

1. The answer is *D*. This patient is postoperative from a laparoscopic sleeve gastrectomy which raises concern for several possible postoperative complications. The gluteal muscle pain on postoperative day zero and the

patient's BMI of greater than 50 g/m² are two of the known associations with developing rhabdomyolysis. The next step in diagnosis requires an elevated creatinine kinase (CK). The CK and serum creatinine should be checked and trended to ensure proper hydration and avoidance of renal failure.

Initiating physical therapy/occupational therapy – Although this is essential in the recovery process, this patient's complaints of gluteal muscle pain immediately postoperatively should raise your suspicion for rhabdomyolysis.

Encouraging incentive spirometry postoperatively is essential in encouraging deep breaths and preventing postoperative atelectasis and pneumonia. This, however, does not present with muscle pain.

Sequential compression boots while the patient is in bed is important in the prevention of deep venous thrombosis in the postoperative patient. Deep venous thrombosis would more likely present with calf pain, not gluteal pain.

2. The answer is *C*. Bariatric equipment is rated for 300–900 pounds of static load.

3. The answer is *A*. Floor-mounted toilets and sinks, as opposed to wall-mounted fixtures, are a very important consideration for the bariatric patient bathroom. The wall-mounted toilets do not have enough capacity to hold the bariatric patient and cause a hazard for the postoperative patient.

Tile flooring may or may not be used in the bariatric bathroom; however, it does not impact the safety of the bariatric patient.

Large bath tubs in the bariatric bathroom would be unsafe as the patient may not be able to maneuver in the tub postoperatively, and it would be difficult for an assistant to help this patient in a bath tub.

Removable shower heads may be convenient in the bariatric bathroom, but they do not impact the safety of this patient.

4. The answer is *False*. This patient's BMI is 45 g/m² which puts him into the category of morbidly obese. These patients require bariatric-rated equipment. Using standard equipment puts the patients as well as the healthcare workers at risk. The bariatric beds are larger for patient comfort, and they are rated for a higher weight. These beds will allow for easier transport and patient transfer as the standard beds will not operate appropriately when the maximum weight limit is exceeded.

5. The answer is *C*. Exquisite tenderness to palpation of the left thigh. Given the lab values above, the potassium is elevated and the creatinine is increased (although we don't have the baseline number, it is not within normal limits). The second clue is the CK level of 5000. Elevated creatinine kinase combined with the elevated creatinine and potassium is concerning for developing kidney injury secondary to rhabdomyolysis. This is a rare complication but can have very serious outcomes if not recognized and treated early. Postoperatively the patients may experience

weakness and muscle fatigue; however, any single area of exquisite tenderness postoperative day one is likely a site of pinpoint pressure intraoperatively and should be monitored closely and reported to the physician caring for the patient.

Pale mucous membranes would correlate with anemia. This patient's hemoglobin is 12.5, which does not raise concern for anemia.

Tachypnea can be seen postoperatively with the most concerning cause being a pulmonary embolus. Nothing in this question stem indicates that this patient is experiencing a pulmonary embolus.

Coarse breath sounds can be a result of atelectasis or developing pneumonia, which are both postoperative complications, especially in the bariatric population. These, however, would likely be reflected by an elevated white count and/or elevated temperature, not an elevated serum creatinine, potassium, or creatinine kinase.

References

1. American Society for Metabolic and Bariatric Surgery (2014) Resources for optimal care of the metabolic and bariatric surgery patient. American College of Surgeons, Chicago
2. Langtree I. Disabled world. 2015. [Online]. Available: http://www.disabled-world.com/. Accessed 7 Feb 2015
3. InPro Corporation (2013) Bariatric design 101. Muskego
4. Chakravartty S, Sarma D, Patel A (2013) Rhabdomyolysis in bariatric surgery: a systematic review. Obes Surg 23(8):1333–1340

Complications of Bariatric Surgery: Gastrointestinal Leak

25

Tatyana Faynberg

Gastrointestinal leak after gastric bypass is a known complication. Its incidence is between 1 and 5 %, and it is associated with a mortality rate of 6–15 % [1]. A leak doubles the risk of mortality and results in a sixfold increase in hospital stay [2]. Patients who develop a leak are at increased risk for wound infection, sepsis, respiratory failure, renal failure, thromboembolism, internal hernia, and small bowel obstruction.

Leaks often present without fever, leukocytosis, or pain. The most common reported symptom of leak is tachycardia; it is present in 72–92 % of patients [3]. There are also studies that report nausea, vomiting, fever, and leukocytosis. A Leak needs to be on the differential diagnosis with any of the symptoms above.

Diagnosis of a leak can be made radiologically or endoscopically. Upper gastrointestinal series with water-soluble contrast and computed tomography (CT) scans have limited sensitivity because of body habitus but high positive predictive value [3]. The weight limitations for CT and MRI scanners in a regular hospital facility range from 135 to 200 kg (300–450 lbs.). CT scanners that can accommodate patients of up to 350 kg body weight (800 lbs) are available but are very expensive and therefore not purchased by most hospitals. For that reason, surgeons performing bariatric surgery should know the weight limitations of the radiology equipment in their facility because some patients are expected to exceed the body weight limitations. Additionally, patient weight has a large effect on enhancement by intravenous contrast material both in the vascular system and in parenchymal organs such as the liver. Nevertheless, computerized tomography of the abdomen after gastric bypass can detect leaks, abscesses, internal hernias, and bowel obstruction. Other limitations of CT are patient positioning and the inability to ingest adequate oral contrast secondary to nausea and vomiting. Because of all of the reasons discussed above,

T. Faynberg, DO
Department of General Surgery, Rowan University, Stratford, NJ, USA
e-mail: faynbeta@rowan.edu

© Springer International Publishing Switzerland 2017
A. Lovcitt ct al. (cds.), *Passing the Certified Bariatric Nurses Exam*,
DOI 10.1007/978-3-319-41703-5_25

CT has not consistently demonstrated a high level of sensitivity in detecting early postoperative leaks.

Upper GI contrast examination is utilized by many surgeons to evaluate the gastro-jejunostomy in patients with suspected leak after gastric bypass. Numerous factors may influence the accuracy of such testing including patient-related factors such as the ability to stand, balance, move about, and swallow and the size of the patient. Sensitivity of upper GI contrast examination varies among reports between 22 and 75 % [3].

When a leak is suspected, endoscopic investigation is warranted. Endoscopic procedures involve the examination of the esophagus, stomach, and gastric pouch (in gastric bypass). During endoscopic examination under fluoroscopy, a bubble test such as submerging the stomach while endoscopically insufflated (bubbles indicate presence of a leak) and injection of contrast with methylene blue into an abdominal drain while looking endoscopically and fluoroscopically for evidence of leak can be performed. These tests are very sensitive for gastric leak [4].

The management of patients with postoperative leak is very challenging because of multiple conditions including the time since the surgical procedure, the type of surgical procedure, and the stability of the patient. Surgical management is associated with high morbidity and mortality. Therefore, initial management is conservative or endoscopic. It begins with supportive care, placing patient nothing by mouth, ordering parenteral or distal enteral feeding, and adding broad-spectrum antibiotics to current medications and percutaneous drainage of any collections found on imaging studies [5].

Endoscopic management is also available. Stent placement for exclusion of the leak from the gastrointestinal tract is the most widely accepted treatment. The stent allows the leak to heal while enteral nutrition is resumed, and it also leads to reduction of peritoneal contamination and improvement in abdominal pain. Common complications of stent placement include chest pain that radiates toward the back, nausea, and stent migration. Stents are usually left in place for 2–8 weeks because longer periods can increase extraction difficulty or can cause stent erosion [4].

Laparoscopic or open re-exploration is an option when gastrointestinal leak is suspected. Re-exploration is characterized by a higher sensitivity, specificity, and accuracy than any other postoperative test to assess for leak and should be considered to be the definitive assessment for the possibility of leak [6]. It is a safe intervention when compared to the consequences of peritonitis, excessive inflammatory response, sepsis, organ failure, and mortality which may develop when diagnosis and treatment of a leak are delayed secondary to false-negative imaging studies. It should be considered in patients with suspected leak, and it is important to note that reliance on false-negative imaging studies may delay operative intervention [6].

Review Questions

1. A 35-year-old female status post gastric sleeve postoperative day 14 without prior medical problems came to the ER because of the increased epigastric abdominal pain. In the ER she has sustained tachycardia in 120 s with blood pressure of 114/65. Her WBC count is 15.5. What is the most likely diagnosis for this patient?

     A. Pulmonary embolism
     B. Gastric leak
     C. Inadequate pain control
     D. Pneumonia
     E. Gastroenteritis

2. The first sign of a gastric leak is:

     A. Tachycardia
     B. Shortness of the breath
     C. Nausea
     D. Right upper quadrant abdominal pain
     E. Mental status change

3. A 55-year-old female developed an anastomotic leak next to gastro-esophageal junction and had a stent endoscopically placed. How long on average she should keep stent in?

     A. 2 days
     B. 2 weeks
     C. 6 days
     D. 6 weeks
     E. 6 months

Answers

1. *B*. The patient has tachycardia accompanied by abdominal pain. Gastric sleeve leak needs to be high on differential as well as PE. With an elevated WBC count of 15.5, the most likely diagnosis is leak.
2. *A*. The first sign of the gastric leak is tachycardia. The presentation is often accompanied by abdominal pain and increase in WBC count.
3. *D*. The stent should be removed at an average of 6 weeks. Longer periods can increase extraction difficulty or can cause stent erosion. Earliest stent removal will not allow the leak to appropriately heal.

References

1. Durak E, Inabnet WB, Schrope B et al (2008) Incidence and management of enteric leaks after gastric bypass for morbid obesity during a 10-year period. Surg Obes Relat Dis 4(5):689
2. Burgos AM, Braghetto I, Csendes A et al (2009) Gastric leak after laparoscopic-sleeve gastrectomy for obesity. Obes Surg 19:1672–1677
3. The American Society for Metabolic and Bariatric Surgery Clinical Issues Committee. Prevention and detection of gastrointestinal leak. ASMBS Executive Council; 2009
4. Kumar N, Thompson CC (2013) Endoscopic management of complications after gastroentestinal weight surgery. Clin Gastroenterol Hepatol 11(4):343–353
5. Csendes A, Burgos AM, Braghetto I (2012) Classification and management of leaks after gastric bypass for patients with morbid obesity: a prospective study of 60 patients. Obes Surg 22:855–862
6. Lee S, Carmody B, Wolfe L et al (2007) Effect of location and speed of diagnosis on anastomotic leak outcomes in 3828 gastric bypass cases. J Gastrointest Surg 11(6):708–713

Complications of Bariatric Surgery: Venous Thromboembolism

26

Tatyana Faynberg

One of the major complications of bariatric surgery is venous thromboembolic (VTE) disease which manifests itself as deep venous thrombosis (DVT) and/or pulmonary embolism (PE). The risk of DVT is between 1 and 3 %, and PE is between 0.2 and 2 % within 30 days of bariatric surgery [1, 2]. While uncommon, PE is one of the leading causes of death within the postoperative period. There are multiple factors that place obese patients at higher risk for VTE [3]:

- Increased body weight by itself is an independent risk for VTE events. It leads to an increased intra-abdominal pressure and decreases venous return to the heart contributing to venous stasis.
- Inactivity causes venous stasis and increased blood viscosity in the lower extremity veins that contributes to the formation of blood clot in the lower extremities.
- Finally, there are also multiple obesity-related biochemical changes that contribute to the increased risk of VTE.

Bariatric surgery further contributes to the already increased risk of VTE events for obese patients [4]:

- Reverse trendelenburg positioning (head of the table up) and pneumoperitoneum (filling the abdomen with CO_2) during surgery decrease venous return to the heart and thus contribute to a prothrombic state.
- Decreased mobility after surgery secondary to pain.

Bariatric surgery patients are considered moderate to high risks of VTE events. Therefore, bariatric centers have implemented multiple VTE protocols. The guidelines for prevention of perioperative VTE events are variable. There are

T. Faynberg, DO
Department of General Surgery, Rowan University, Stratford, NJ, USA
e-mail: faynbeta@rowan.edu

© Springer International Publishing Switzerland 2017
A. Loveitt et al. (eds.), *Passing the Certified Bariatric Nurses Exam*,
DOI 10.1007/978-3-319-41703-5_26

115

multiple accepted forms for DVT prevention such as mechanical compression devices, early ambulation, chemoprophylaxis, and sometimes the use of inferior vena cava filters (IVC). The majority of the bariatric surgeons routinely use (1) early ambulation, (2) pharmacologic agents, and (3) mechanical compression devices to prevent VTE complications. The most commonly used chemical agents are unfractionated heparin or enoxaparin [4, 5].

Heparin works by binding to the enzyme inhibitor antithrombin III (ATIII). It activates thrombin (factor IIa) and factor Xa. Heparin is reversible and has a short half-life. Prophylactic dosing of 5000 units every 8–12 h is common. The most serious side effect is heparin-induced thrombocytopenia (HIT). HIT is an antibody-mediated attack on platelets and can lead to significant bleeding as the platelet level drops. It is treated by discontinuation of all heparin products and starting other means of chemoprophylaxis.

Lovenox (low molecular weight heparin) is another popular chemoprophylactic agent among bariatric surgeons. It acts mostly on factor Xa. It requires less frequent administration and significantly lower risk of HIT, but compared to heparin, it is more expensive and the half-life is longer. Additionally it is not as easily reversible.

Inferior vena cava filters (IVCFs) are mechanical devices that trap venous thromboembolism that originates in lower extremities and can go to the lungs. They are usually placed into high-risk patients who have known hypercoagulable state, prior history of VTE, or very high BMI.

The most common complaint of a patient with a suspected DVT is lower extremity pain [2]. While physical exam of the lower extremities is limited in the morbidly obese, you should look for swelling of the lower extremity, tenderness over the calf area, discoloration of the skin, or a palpable cord On physical exam, you can find swelling of the lower extremity, tenderness over the calf area, discoloration of the skin, or palpable cord. The most common modality used to evaluate for DVT is ultrasound of lower extremities. Ultrasound is noninvasive and has greater than 95 % sensitivity and specificity for proximal DVT. Findings suggestive of DVT on ultrasound will be noncompressibility of the vein and abnormal flow within the vein.

PE most commonly manifests itself as dyspnea on exertion, chest pain, decrease in oxygen saturation, and tachycardia. Signs such as tachypnea, decreased breath sounds, unilateral lower extremity pain, and hypotension may also be found. In jugular venous distention, the presence of the right-sided S3 heart sound can be seen in massive PE because of right heart strain. The most commonly used modality to confirm the presence of PE is an ABG and a spiral CT. Less commonly ordered studies include a pulmonary angiography and ventilation/perfusion (V/Q) scan.

Treatment for PE and DVT is therapeutic anticoagulation. Although obtaining confirmatory studies is always preferred, if there is a high suspicion for PE and the patient is hemodynamically unstable, empiric administration of anticoagulation may be necessary. Documented VTE should be treated with long-term anticoagulation for 3–6 months. Most commonly the patient is transitioned to oral warfarin with a goal INR between 2.0 and 3.0. Indications for the use of IVC filters in the setting of PE are high risk of bleeding, PE despite being on anticoagulation, and thromboembolic burden that can cause further propagation of the clot.

1. If chemoprophylaxis is not used in the perioperative bariatric surgery setting, what other strategies can be employed to decrease VTE risk?

   A. Early ambulation after surgery
   B. Mechanical device prophylaxis
   C. A and B
   D. Placing patient on bed rest
   E. Starting vitamin supplementation sooner

2. What are the known DVT risks?

   A. Immobility
   B. Venous stasis
   C. Endothelial injury
   D. A, B, and C are correct
   E. Early ambulation

3. A 45-year-old female just underwent a gastric sleeve, her postoperative course was complicated by uncontrolled pain, and she refuses to ambulate. She has now started to complain of the pain in her right calf. What is your study of choice to confirm patient's condition?

   A. Right lower extremity ultrasound
   B. Bilateral lower extremities CT scan
   C. Right lower extremity x-ray
   D. Cardiac stress test
   E. Bilateral lower extremity arterial Dopplers

4. A 54-year-old male with a BMI of 45 status post laparoscopic Roux-en-Y gastric bypass is now postoperative day 3. He develops sudden onset of chest pain and is persistently tachycardic 120 s with complaints of shortness of breath. While examining the patient, you note that he is not talking in full sentences and his O2 saturation is 65%. What is the next step in taking care of this patient?

   A. Address patient's airway first.
   B. Send patient to CT angiogram of the chest STAT.
   C. Give patient warfarin STAT.
   D. Call pharmacy for heparin drip.
   E. Send patient for CT scan of abdomen pelvis; he probably has a leak.

1. The answer is C. If chemoprophylaxis is not used in the perioperative bariatric surgery setting, patients should be instructed to start ambulating early and have compression devices on lower extremities every time the patient is in bed. Placing the patient on bed rest will cause patient to be immobile and thus contribute to DVT. Starting vitamins has nothing to do with VTE prophylaxis.

2. The answer is *D*. Immobility, venous stasis, and endothelial injury are contributors to developing a DVT. Early ambulation is a preventative measure.

3. The answer is *A*. The most likely diagnosis is DVT and ultrasound is the test of choice. CT scan, x-ray, and *arterial* Dopplers play no role in the diagnosis of DVT although they may help in the diagnosis of less common causes of lower extremity pain. A cardiac stress test has no role in this situation.

4. The answer is *A*. Anytime a patient is in significant respiratory distress, the airway should be addressed first, and this patient likely requires intubation. The most probable diagnosis in this case is massive PE, and CT angiogram should be performed when the patient is stable for transfer.

References

1. Rocha AT, de Vasconcellos AG, da Luz Neto ER et al (2006) Risk of venous thromboembolism and efficacy of thromboprophylaxis in hospitalized obese medical patients and in obese patients undergoing bariatric surgery. Obes Surg 16:1645–1655
2. Winegar DA, Sherif B, Pate V, DeMaria EJ (2011) Venous thromboembolism after bariatric surgery performed by Bariatric Surgery Center of Excellence Participants: analysis of the Bariatric Outcomes Longitudinal Database. Surg Obes Relat Dis 7:181–188
3. Stein PD, Beemath A, Olson RE (2005) Obesity as a risk factor in venous thromboembolism. Am J Med 118:978–980
4. Bartlett MA, Mauck KF, Daniels PR; Division of General Internal Medicine, Mayo Clinic Thrombophilia Center. Prevention of venous thromboembolism in bariatric surgery patients. Mayo Clinic, Rochester; 2015
5. Freeman AL, Pendleton RC, Rondina MT (2010) Prevention of venous thromboembolism in obesity. Expert Rev Cardiovasc Ther 8(12):1711–1721

Complications of Bariatric Surgery: Obstruction

27

Tatyana Faynberg

Bowel obstruction is a very rare complication of sleeve gastrectomy and laparoscopic adjustable gastric banding but has been reported to have an overall incidence of up to 5 % in patients after laparoscopic Roux-en-Y gastric bypass (LRYGB) [1]. Similar to other types of bowel obstruction, patients present with abdominal pain, nausea and vomiting, and minimal or no bowel function.

Diagnosis of small bowel obstructions is made clinically, and with the help of CT scans, small bowel follows through or upper GI series. Causes of obstructions such as internal hernias can be missed on the imaging studies and present with vague symptoms, so there should be a very low threshold for taking the patient to the operating room.

Obstructions can be early or late. Early post-operative small bowel obstructions tend to result from technical problems with the Roux limb and require revision of the bypass or small bowel resection [2]. Early small bowel obstructions are more frequently treated operatively than late obstructions. Also, in the very immediate postoperative period, acute stenosis at the gastrojejunal anastomosis may develop secondary to surrounding tissue edema. In these cases, nasogastric decompression and bowel rest may be helpful until resolution of the edema and stenosis occurs. It is very important to properly diagnose technical problems because they can cause grave consequences for the patient if not fixed in timely manner.

Etiologies of late small bowel obstruction include adhesions, internal hernias, abdominal wall hernias, and intussusceptions [3]. Adhesions are most commonly seen after open gastric bypass surgery. Internal hernias are more frequently seen after laparoscopic procedures and have an incidence of 3–16 % [4]. They occur when portions of the small bowel slip through defects in the mesentery created during surgery. This results in obstruction of the blood supply and ischemia. They are extremely difficult to diagnose because of nonspecific symptoms such as cramping,

T. Faynberg, DO
Department of General Surgery, Rowan University, Stratford, NJ, USA
e-mail: faynbeta@rowan.edu

© Springer International Publishing Switzerland 2017
A. Loveitt et al. (eds.), *Passing the Certified Bariatric Nurses Exam*,
DOI 10.1007/978-3-319-41703-5_27

periumbilical pain, nausea, and vomiting. Also diagnostic radiographic studies can be normal, or have very subtle findings such as mesenteric edema or englarged mesenteric lymph nodes. Low threshold for re-exploration is indicated in bariatric patients with unexplained pain or symptoms of bowel obstruction because internal hernias sometimes can be missed on radiologic studies.

Incisional hernias were reported to be the most frequent late complication in open gastric bypass, occurring in 8.6–20 % of patients [1]. In the era of laparoscopic surgery, this is drastically less.

Intussusception, or telescoping of the bowel, is a rare late complication after gastric bypass with an incidence of about 1 % [2]. It can present several years after surgery and most often occurs in women after significant weight loss. The etiology is not well understood but appears to be multifactorial, involving a lead point such as suture lines, adhesions, or motility disturbances from the ectopic pacemaker development that occurs with the change in anatomy. Management can be laparoscopic or open exploration to reduce the intussusception, but frequently requires resection and reconstruction of the involved segment of bowel.

Review Questions

1. What are the causes of early small bowel obstructions?

   A. Internal hernia
   B. Adhesions
   C. Anastomotic edema
   D. Technical problems
   E. C and D

2. What are the symptoms of small bowel obstructions?

   A. Nausea
   B. Vomiting
   C. Loss of bowel function
   D. Abdominal pain
   E. All of the above

3. What are the late causes of small bowel obstructions in bariatric patients?

   A. Internal hernias
   B. Tissue Edema
   C. Adhesions
   D. Technical problems
   E. A and C

Answers

1. The answer is *E*. Technical problems and anastomotic edema are the early causes of small bowel obstructions in bariatric patients. Technical problem should be always on the back mind since failure to recognize it can have grave consequences for the patient.

2. The answer is *E*. Proximally to the obstruction are caused by the blockage of the small bowel, gastric contents back up proximally to obstruction and cause the patient to vomit. This also results in loss of outflow including bowel movements and gas. As the obstruction becomes worse, the patient may experience pain both from distention of the bowel and, in severe cases, peritoneal inflammation.

3. The answer is *E*. Internal hernias tend to occur late, especially after a patient has lost a significant amount of weight which acts to enlarge the mesenteric defect. Adhesions can also develop and lead to obstruction. Technical problems and tissue edema tend to present early in the postoperative course.

References

1. Husain S, Ahmed AR, Johnson J, Boss T, O'Malley W (2007) Small-bowel obstruction after laparoscopic Roux-en-Y gastric bypass: etiology, diagnosis, and management. Arch Surg 142(10):988–993
2. Hwang RF, Swartz DE, Felix EL (2004) Causes of small bowel obstruction after laparoscopic gastric bypass. Surg Endosc 18(11):1631–1635
3. Rogula T, Yenumula PR, Schauer PR (2007) A complication of Roux-en-Y gastric bypass: intestinal obstruction. Surg Endosc 21(11):1914–1918
4. Steele KE, Prokopowicz GP, Magnuson T, Lidor A, Schweitzer M (2008) Laparoscopic antecolic Roux-en-Y gastric bypass with closure of internal defects leads to fewer internal hernias than the retrocolic approach. Surg Endosc 22(9):2056–2061

Complications of Bariatric Surgery: Dehydration

28

Lynn J. Stott

The power of education for the preoperative bariatric patient can never be underestimated and can help prevent complications. With the limited length of the hospital stay, it is critical that all future bariatric patients are thoroughly informed on how to prepare for surgery, their hospital experience, and diet stages, how to recognize the basic needs of their bodies, and how to prevent complications. Nurses as well as medical staff should be sensitive to the potential lack of healthcare literacy and language barriers when educating bariatric patients. Furthermore, the entire clinical staff on the bariatric unit should receive updated bariatric education and continuing education courses annually to assure that they are giving the best possible care to the postoperative patients as well as recognizing complications early [1].

There are many potential bariatric postoperative complications, but one that is most likely preventable pertains to dehydration. Dehydration occurs when the body loses too much fluid. Signs and symptoms of dehydration include thirst, decrease in skin turgor, dry or cool skin, dry mucous membranes, constipation, low or minimal urine output, muscle cramps, tachycardia, hypotension, light-headedness, feeling dizzy, headache, fever, nausea, malaise, diaphoresis, irritability, confusion, and, in serious cases, delirium or loss of consciousness.

Postoperative monitoring of bariatric patients has revealed a large number of these patients require 1–3 l of intravenous fluid boluses to maintain adequate hydration. Furthermore, patients may have difficulty voiding, or a urine output of <100 mL per void with a foul odor and often a dark amber color. How can we prevent this?

All patients should undergo a bariatric preoperative education class. The topic of dehydration should be emphasized as a preventable complication. Patients may already be in a state of dehydration prior to arriving on their scheduled surgical day; thus, the education should be enhanced to include the following information [1]:

L.J. Stott, RN, CMSRN, CBN
Kennedy University Hospital, 18 East Laurel Road, Stratford, NJ 08084, USA
e-mail: L.Stott@kennedyhealth.org

© Springer International Publishing Switzerland 2017   123
A. Loveitt et al. (eds.), *Passing the Certified Bariatric Nurses Exam*,
DOI 10.1007/978-3-319-41703-5_28

1. The patient should be instructed to drink plenty of fluids the day before surgery, resulting in increased urination and light yellow to clear appearance of their urine.
2. A majority of patients have been found to have a lack of healthcare literacy and/ or language barriers. The class information should visually reflect what the 64 ounces (almost 2 l) daily fluid requirement looks like by showing eight 8 ounce cups (240 ml) of fluid. Also the presentation should review the signs and symptoms of dehydration in simple terms.
3. A "urine color chart" should be placed in all the bariatric bathrooms, as well as in their gift bags for home, to remind the patient to drink enough fluids, resulting in urine that will look light yellow to clear in appearance.
4. It is challenging to reach the goal of 64 ounces of fluid per day due to the small stomach pouch limiting the stomach capacity to accept fluids. Also, patients should be taught the 30/30 rule, meaning they do not ingest fluids 30 min before a meal and wait 30 min after meals to prevent gastrointestinal symptoms and feelings of fullness. Consequently, patients can be instructed to start drinking early in the day, to sip fluids continuously during their waking hours, and to carry a beverage or sports drink with them at all times. They can be taught to be mindful if they are exercising or perspiring during warmer days, because the risk of dehydration quickly increases.
5. Beverages to avoid include carbonated drinks because they cause discomfort to the stomach. Caffeine should also be avoided because it can interfere with calcium absorption leading to a deficiency and is also considered a mild diuretic.

The clinical nurse's role starts with preoperative education and support on the patient's weight loss journey. By having a well-hydrated bariatric patient prior to surgery, it is possible to avoid the complication of dehydration postoperatively. Education and visual instruction can potentially decrease the number of hospital readmissions related to dehydration.

Review Questions

1. A 47-year-old Hispanic female arrives to the ER, postoperative bariatric surgery day 4. She states that she "just does not feel good, has nausea, light-headedness, and headache." She does not remember the last time she voided. Upon assessment, the nurse discovers that the patient did not attend the bariatric preoperative class due to her job demands and she speaks and reads minimal English. Her BP is 89/40, HR 120, and temperature 98.8. What is most likely her diagnosis?

   A. Gastric leak
   B. Dumping syndrome
   C. Dehydration
   D. Acute renal failure

2. The ER nurse obtains STAT lab studies for the patient above. What would be their next priority?

    A. Have the patient drink a glass of water.
    B. Weigh the patient.
    C. Walk the patient to the bathroom to obtain a urine sample.
    D. Start IVF bolus of NSS with a doctor order.

3. The patient appears very upset and confused. She does not seem to understand everything the medical staff is telling her because she keeps answering "yes" to all questions. What is the underlying problem?

    A. The patient is confused due to her symptoms.
    B. The patient is worried that she is going to be readmitted to the hospital.
    C. The medical staff is not being sensitive to the patient's healthcare illiteracy and the language line should be utilized.
    D. The patient is being difficult.

4. The patient was admitted to the surgical unit on a telemetry monitor, remains in bed for over 24 h, and voids on the bedpan. Her HR is 109, BP 98/60, and temperature 101.2. The lung sounds show rhonchi at the bases. What does the nurse suspect is occurring?

    A. Septic shock
    B. Gastric Leak
    C. Pneumonia related to inactivity and not utilizing the incentive spirometer hourly
    D. Noncompliance of the patient to get out of the bed

5. After remaining in the hospital for 48 h of treatment with IV fluids and IV antibiotics, the stage II bariatric diet was introduced, and the patient improved enough to return home on oral antibiotics. The nurse educates the patient using the language line on all of the following *except*:

    A. Continue on the stage II bariatric diet, and on your follow-up doctor visit, they will tell you when to advance to the stage III diet.
    B. Set a goal to lose at least 20 pounds this month.
    C. No drinking fluids 30 min before meals and 30 min after meals.
    D. Avoid drinking caffeine beverages such as coffee right now.

Answers

1. The answer is *C*. The patient has classic symptoms of dehydration including oliguria, tachycardia, hypotension, nausea, headache, and lightheadedness. The patient does not have abdominal pain or a fever as a combination of the above symptoms, so it does not appear to be a gastric leak. No labs were obtained yet to suspect ARF, and the patient is on the stage I diet, so it does not support dumping syndrome.

2. The answer is *D*. The patient needs IV fluid replacement due to dehydration and may not be able to take oral fluids due to nausea. The nurse should continue to monitor HR and BP plus the time and volume of any urine output. The patient's weight is not a priority, and walking the patient while they feel lightheaded is a safety issue.
3. The answer is *C*. Healthcare illiteracy is evident in a large majority of patients. Education, using simple terms and visual aids, is crucial in helping the patient understand their body's needs. Staff cannot assume that the patient is confused or difficult especially if English is not their primary language. It is every patient's right to have the language line or hospital-approved interpreter available so that communication is clear and understandable.
4. The answer is *C*. There has to be at least two specific factors to meet the septic shock diagnosis, so this cannot be the answer. The first classic symptom of a gastric leak is tachycardia, specifically an HR >120, and this patient has a HR of 109. One cannot assume that the patient is non-compliant as this would be judging without any evidence. The complication of pneumonia can possibly be avoided by early ambulation and the use of the pulmonary toilet (incentive spirometer, coughing with a splint pillow, and deep breathing).
5. The answer is *B*. Setting specific time-related weight loss goals is not suggested and can be very psychologically defeating to the patient. The emphasis during the initial 4 weeks postsurgery is about healing and adjusting to a new lifestyle. The doctor or their staff will instruct the patient when it is time to advance to the next diet stage. The 30/30 rule is used so the patient can eat their diet without feeling full too quickly, and caffeine can dehydrate the bariatric patient, so it is avoided initially.

Reference

1. Mechanick J, Youdim A, Jones D et al (2013) Clinical practice guidelines for the perioperative nutritional, metabolic, and nonsurgical support of the bariatric patient – 2013 update. Surg Obes Relat Dis 9:159–191

Nasogastric Tube Placement in the Bariatric Patient

Rahul Sharma

The nasogastric tubes (NGTs) are a commonly used instrument in the field of surgery. Most NGTs are single- or double-lumen tubes made of flexible plastic which are inserted through the nasal passageways down the throat and into the stomach. Measured markings and standardized techniques allow for the blind insertion of NGTs on a routine basis by physicians and nurses. NGTs are used to decompress the stomach, remove gastric contents in the case of a blockage, and also administer medications or feeding in patients unable to swallow on their own.

In the case of postoperative bariatric patients, routine NGT placement is *not* recommended [1]. The gastric anatomy is drastically different from normal, and a fresh staple line is vulnerable to direct trauma leading to a leak. This presents a quandary for providers as nausea, vomiting, and postoperative ileus are known complications after bariatric surgery and are often treated with NGT placement in non-bariatric surgery patients. If absolutely necessary, NGTs may be placed by a physician or designee. They must be extremely gentle, stop at the first sign of resistance, and preferably place the tube under direct visualization, such as using upper endoscopy.

Even after a bariatric surgery patient's staple line has healed, they should not undergo blind NGT insertion unless it is an absolute emergency. Normal gastric anatomy is forgiving when an overly long NGT is inserted, as the tube simply coils in the stomach and continues to function. In a gastric sleeve or Roux-en-Y patient, the tube does not have enough room to turn and can damage or perforate the stomach, leading to leakage of contents into the abdominal cavity and emergent need for surgery [2]. Some bariatric centers provide patients with a medical alert-type bracelet which instructs prehospital and hospital personnel not to blindly insert NGTs.

Finally, when NGTs are inserted and portable x-rays are used to verify placement, the radiologist and staff should be informed of the patient's bariatric surgery

R. Sharma, DO, MPH
Department of General Surgery, Rowan University, Stratford, NJ, USA
e-mail: sharmar6@rowan.edu

© Springer International Publishing Switzerland 2017   127
A. Loveitt et al. (eds.), *Passing the Certified Bariatric Nurses Exam*,
DOI 10.1007/978-3-319-41703-5_29

history [3]. Case reports exist where patients had gastric perforations from NGTs, and the radiologists did not identify them due to the lack of information on the patient's altered anatomy [2]. The patient's post-bariatric status should be included in every shift sign out as well as when ordering tests.

Review Questions

1. A patient presents to the emergency department complaining of nausea and intractable vomiting. They underwent an uncomplicated sleeve gastrectomy 2 weeks prior. Which of the following is the best first step in patient care?

   A. Tell the patient this is a normal side effect of the surgery.
   B. Insert an NGT and place on low intermittent suction.
   C. Notify the surgical team and manage the patient's symptoms medically.
   D. Intubate the patient to prevent aspiration.
   E. Obtain an x-ray as the patient likely has a staple line leak

2. You insert a routine NGT into a patient with a likely small bowel obstruction. You aspirate what appears to be gastric contents. After a short time, the patient's family informs you that they underwent a Roux-en-Y bypass years ago. What is your next action?

   A. Immediately remove the NGT.
   B. Call the surgical team to evaluate the patient.
   C. Order an abdominal x-ray to evaluate tube placement.
   D. Stop using the tube for suction and for administering medications.
   E. B, C, and D.

3. Which of the following is the most correct reason for not blindly placing an NGT in a postoperative bariatric patient?

   A. The smaller gastric anatomy makes the tip of the NGT induce nausea and vomiting
   B. The altered gastric anatomy makes the semirigid NGT difficult to advance into the proper position.
   C. The tip of the NGT may perforate staple lines in the stomach even if they have been healed for a long time.
   D. Nausea and vomiting in a postoperative bariatric patient can always be managed with medication.
   E. None of the above.

4. You are providing discharge instructions to a postoperative Roux-en-Y patient when they ask you about NGTs. They heard from a friend that they should NEVER have an NGT placed and they should go as far as refuse treatment if one is offered. How should you counsel your patient?

   A. Agree with the patient and their friend. Refusing NGT and any associated treatment is appropriate and prudent.

B. Counsel the patient to inform any medical providers they are being treated by that they have had bariatric surgery. In some cases, NGTs are appropriate if placed carefully.
C. Counsel the patient that as long as the NGT is shorter than normal, it may be placed if needed.
D. Counsel the patient that they will never need an NGT as their symptoms can always be managed medically.

Answers

1. The answer is *C*. Nausea and vomiting is a common side effect of the surgery; however, it could also be the start of something more serious. NGTs should not be inserted blindly unless it is an emergency. This patient should be managed medically until the surgical team can decide whether an NGT is necessary or not.
2. The answer is *E*. The tube may be in the correct position, but with the patient's altered anatomy, you should check its placement. An x-ray will help confirm that the tube is within the stomach. The surgical team will help you evaluate placement. Until the tube is confirmed, you should not use it for anything.
3. The answer is *C*. Blindly advancing an NGT may cause it to become lodged in and then perforate a staple line as it does not have room to turn and coil on itself in a postoperative bariatric patient. *A* and *B* are partially correct but are not the most important reason for not blindly placing a tube.
4. The answer is *B*. Refusing NGT in all circumstances (*A*) would not be wise, as the patient may need one in the future if they ever develop a bowel obstruction. *C* is incorrect as blind tube insertion, no matter what length, could lead to perforation. *D* is incorrect as you do not know what medical problems the patient may develop in the distant future. Immediate postoperative nausea/vomiting is very easily controlled with medication, but this does not preclude future issues such as bowel obstruction.

References

1. Thompson C. Ask the expert: endoscopy in the bariatric patient. *ASGE News,* Nov 2010
2. Van Dinter TG, John L, Guileyardo JM, John SF (2013) Intestinal perforation caused by insertion of a nasogastric tube late after gastric bypass. Proc Baylor Univ Med Cent 26(1):11–15
3. Luber SD, Fischer DR, Venkat A (2008) Care of the bariatric patient in the emergency department. J Emerg Med 34(1):13–20

Pharmacologic Considerations in Obesity

30

Mara Piltin

Pharmaceutical drug administration can be a very complex science in the obese population. Recommended medication doses are based on normal-weight patients, which can make dosing difficult when considering the physiologic changes related to both obesity and weight loss surgery. Studies have suggested that increased fat deposition can potentially affect the drug elimination and distribution. There are multiple different ways to describe a patient's weight. These include total body weight (TBW), ideal body weight (IBW), adjusted body weight (ABW), and lean body mass (LBM) [1].

Total body weight (TBW) = patient's actual weight

Ideal Body Weight (IBW)
Males: IBW (kg) = 50 kg + 2.3 kg per every inch over 5 ft
Females: IBW (kg) = 45.5 kg + 2.3 kg per every inch over 5 ft

Adjusted body weight (ABW) = IBW + 0.4 (actual weight – IBW)
*ABW is only used if the actual body weight is >30 % of the calculated IBW.

Lean Body Mass (LBM)
Male: LBM = 1.1(weight) -128(weight/height)^2
Female: LBM = 1.07(weight) -148(weight/height)^2

Many pharmacologic parameters used to describe medications can vary in the obese patient. These include volume of distribution, clearance, and protein binding. The volume of distribution of substances that are highly lipophilic (fat loving) may be significantly increased in the obese population, e.g., benzodiazepines and barbiturates [1].

M. Piltin, DO
Department of General Surgery, Rowan University, Stratford, NJ, USA
e-mail: piltinma@rowan.edu

© Springer International Publishing Switzerland 2017
A. Loveitt et al. (eds.), *Passing the Certified Bariatric Nurses Exam*,
DOI 10.1007/978-3-319-41703-5_30

131

It has been suggested that obesity can alter the elimination and tissue distribution of medications as well. Maintenance and loading doses of specific medications that require narrow therapeutic windows may need adjustments in the obese population. In bariatric patients, this is an important consideration regarding antibiotics [2]. In a normal-weight individual, the blood flow in fat accounts for only 5 % of the cardiac output. The remaining output is distributed as 22 % to the lean tissue and 73 % to the viscera [3]. Increase in fatty tissue may therefore result in modified hemodynamics and pharmacokinetics of specific medications.

One other consideration to make is that many drugs are metabolized by cytochrome P450. This is a system of enzymes from the liver that function in biotransformation and oxidation of some drugs. Obese patients frequently have fatty deposition in their livers which may alter drug metabolism in a way that is not yet fully understood [2, 4]. Unfortunately, this area of research is still underdeveloped and requires more investigation before definitive recommendations on dosing in obesity can be made.

Some medications do have recommended weight adjustment parameters that we can use for dosing [1, 5]:

Vancomycin – TBW
Ciprofloxacin – IBW + 0.45(excess body weight)
Perioperative cefazolin – increased dose for higher TBW
Lithium – IBW

With regard to drug absorption, the proximal fourth of the intestines accounts for half of the total mucosal surface of the gut. This portion also has the greatest capacity for absorption. When considering Roux-en-Y gastric bypass surgery, there are both restrictive and malabsorptive components of weight loss. This could result in decreased bioavailability of drugs that have delayed absorption. Reducing the stomach to a pouch causes decreased hydrochloric acid production and therefore slightly higher pH. Medications that depend upon gastric ionization may be altered as well [6].

It is well studied that there are improvements and even resolution of some medical conditions after bariatric surgery. These include diseases such as hypertension, hyperlipidemia, asthma, and diabetes. Approximately 70–80 % of post-bypass patients can expect complete remission of type 2 diabetes, hypertension, and hyperlipidemia. It is important to consider postoperative dose adjustments in medications for such conditions. This is relevant in both the immediate postoperative period and the weeks, months, and years to follow. Immediately, there is a drastic shift in the patient's diet with the potential for dehydration and hypoglycemic events. Avoidance of diuretics and decreased insulin doses are recommended postoperatively. As time passes and the body adjusts to weight loss, medication requirements and doses should again be reconsidered on a patient to patient basis [7, 8].

Review Questions

1. What is the calculated ideal body weight (IBW) for a 100 kg woman who is 5 ft 5 in?

   A. 60
   B. 56
   C. 62
   D. 57

2. Perioperative cefazolin dose should be based on which of the following?

   A. Ideal body weight (IBW)
   B. Total body weight (TBW)
   C. Adjusted body weight (ABW)
   D. Lean body mass (LBM)

3. What physiologic changes associated with Roux-en-Y gastric bypass surgery could potentially affect medication doses?

   A. Decreased cardiac output
   B. Decreased gastric hydrochloric acid production
   C. Decreased intestinal absorption
   D. B and C

4. What are the distributions of cardiac output described in this chapter?

   A. 5% fat, 22% lean tissue, 73%-viscera
   B. 10% fat, 20% lean tissue, 70%-viscera
   C. 7% fat, 30% lean tissue, 63% viscera
   D. 2% fat, 30% lean tissue, 68% viscera

Answers

1. The answer is *C*. Using the equation to calculate IBW for females: IBW (kg)=45.5 kg+2.3 kg per every inch over 5 ft. This patient has 5 in over 5 ft which would be 11.5 added to the standard 45.5 kg for females. This results in a value of 62 kg.
2. The answer is *B*. Studies have shown that perioperative cefazolin should be increased from 1 to 2 g depending upon the total body weight of the patient. This is based on a study that illustrated a decreased rate of surgical wound infection in obese patients when cefazolin dose was increased from 1 to 2 g. Some recommend using 2 g for a weight >100 kg or a BMI >30, but these exact parameters are still controversial.
3. The answer is *D*. Decreased hydrochloric acid is a result of creating the stomach into a small pouch. Because of this, the patient is left with fewer acid-producing cells. This may affect medications that require ionization. Decreased intestinal absorption is also a physiologic change related to Roux-en-Y gastric bypass surgery as the small intestines are cut by

45–150 cm from the stomach and re-routed. Decreased cardiac output is not related to Roux-en-Y bypass surgery.
4. The answer is *A*. Cardiac output distributions described here are 5 % fat, 22 % lean tissue, and 73 % viscera.

References

1. De Beardemaeker L, Mortier E, Struys M (2004) Pharmacokinetics in obese patients. Contin Educ Anaesth Crit Care Pain 4:152–155
2. Cheymol G (2000) Effects of obesity on pharmacokinetics implications for drug therapy. Clin Pharmacokinet 39(3):215–233
3. Rowland M, Tozer TN (1995) Clinical pharmacokinetics: concepts and applications. Williams & Wilkins, Baltimore
4. Diehl AM (1999) Nonalcoholic steatohepatitis. Semin Liver Dis 19:221–229
5. Wurtz R, Itokazu G, Rodvold K (1997) Antimicrobial dosing in obese patients. Clin Infect Dis 25:112–118
6. Linares C, Decleves X, Oppert J et al (2009) Pharmacology of morphine in obese patients. Clin Pharmacokinet 48(10):635–651
7. Schauer P, Kashyap S, Wolski K et al (2012) Bariatric surgery versus intensive medical therapy in obese patients with diabetes. N Engl J Med 366(17):1567–1576
8. Tuck M, Sowers J, Dornfeld L, Kledzik G, Maxwell M (1981) The effect of weight reduction on blood pressure, plasma renin activity, and plasma aldosterone levels in obese patients. N Engl J Med 304(16):930–933

Basic Nutrition in Obese Patients

Alyssa Luning and Cheri Leahy

Nutrition by definition is the process of providing or obtaining the food necessary for health and growth. There are many components of nutrition that play a large role in the care of a bariatric patient before and after surgery to support success [1]. Comprehension of how the body accesses and utilizes these nutrients is invaluable in order to encourage appropriate dietary recommendations. The foundation of nutrition for essential human life may be broken down as follows.

31.1 Macronutrients

A substance required in relatively large amounts by living organisms. The body is able to run most efficiently in cell growth, repair, and function throughout all systems when it is provided with the following macronutrients through diet.

31.1.1 Protein

Energy 4 kcal/g

Function Carry out the work of the living cell by serving as enzymes, receptors, transporters, hormones, antibodies, and communicators.

A. Luning, RDN (✉) • C. Leahy, RDN
Kennedy Health Alliance, 2201 Chapel Ave W #100, Cherry Hill, NJ 08002, USA
e-mail: a.luning@kennedyhealth.org; cherileahyrd@gmail.com

© Springer International Publishing Switzerland 2017   135
A. Lovcitt ct al. (eds.), *Passing the Certified Bariatric Nurses Exam*,
DOI 10.1007/978-3-319-41703-5_31

Table 31.1 The essential amino acids

Histidine
Isoleucine
Leucine
Lysine
Methionine plus cystine
Phenylalanine plus tyrosine
Threonine
Tryptophan
Valine

Components

Amino acids linked by peptide bonds. There are 20 amino acids required by humans. There are nonessential amino acids which are produced in the body and 9 essential amino acids which must come from the diet (Table 31.1).

Examples in patient care:

- Patients are typically given a daily high protein gram intake goal to assist in healing and repair after surgery. Daily intake goals may range anywhere from 60 to 80 g for women and 80–100 g for men.
- This may vary by the individual if there are any compromising health concerns related to a high-protein diet (such as with kidney disease).
- Protein recommendations may range from 1.2 to 1.5 g per kilogram of a patient's ideal body weight down to .8–1 g per kilogram of a patient's ideal body weight.
- Higher protein diets in patients after bariatric surgery are recommended to promote healing for 1–3 months after surgery. After this time, patients' needs should be assessed via routine lab work, if possible lean body mass analysis, and patient interview to determine if it is still medically necessary to maintain a high-protein diet.
- If a patient is unable to maintain their high-protein diet, they are at greater risk for decreased rate of healing, fatigue, lethargy, protein-calorie malnutrition, and hair loss.
- A good bariatric team should provide the patient with information, resources, and tips on how to accurately keep track of protein intake. It is the patient's responsibility after their procedure to make an effort to meet their dietary goals.
- Before and after surgery, patients are typically instructed to navigate the market for protein supplements to increase protein intake while still using smaller portion sizes. They are recommended to use these protein supplements in shakes and to add them into foods such as yogurts, puddings, or hot cereal.
- It is important for patients to find powders that are complete proteins (including all amino acids), <5 g of sugar per serving and somewhere between 15 and 30 g of protein per serving for optimum absorption [2]. The most popular varieties are whey protein isolate and plant-based protein powders (such as blends of pea, brown rice, and hemp). These are best tolerated, easy to find over the counter and are both popular and nutrient dense sources of complete protein to prepare for, and to heal after surgery.

Table 31.2 Popular dietary sources of lean protein (per ounce)

Tuna (canned): 7 g
Chicken (cooked): 4 g
Greek yogurt (nonfat): 3 g
Tofu (extra firm): 3 g
Lentils (cooked): 3 g

- If a patient is not amendable to using a protein supplement to increase their intake, they typically use alternative methods of increasing protein intake, such as adding things like nonfat dried milk powder, egg whites, silken tofu, plain Greek yogurt, and other low-fat dairy foods into their diet (Table 31.2).
- A caution on exceeding protein gram recommendations: patients who exceed recommendations on daily protein intake may be at increased risk for constipation, stress on the kidney or other organs, dehydration, hypertension, and high LDL cholesterol. Current research does not support any evidence that excessive protein intake is beneficial for weight loss or weight loss maintenance.

31.1.2 Fat

Energy 9 kcal/g

Function Fats/lipids constitute 34 % of the energy in the human diet [1]. Stored in adipose cells, humans are able to survive for weeks and months if there is little or no food available. The fat not used effectively is called structural fat which pads organs and nerves in position to protect them against injury, protects bones from mechanical pressure, and even insulates the body. Fat in the diet is essential for digestion and absorption of fat-soluble vitamins and phytochemicals.

Components

- Fatty Acids: simple lipids (neutral fats + waxes)
- Saturated fatty acid: no double bonds between carbons
- Monounsaturated fatty acids: one double bond
- Polyunsaturated fatty acids: two or more double bonds
- Essential Fatty Acids: must be consumed by the diet and cannot be synthesized in the human body alone. Optimum ratio is 2:1–3:1 for brain health
- Omega-6: arachidonic acid (ALA) – flaxseed, canola, soybean oils, and some green leafy vegetables
- Omega-3: eicosapentaenoic acid (EPA) – cod liver oil, mackerel, salmon, sardines, and sea vegetables
- Compound lipids: phospholipids, glycolipids, and lipoproteins
- Miscellaneous lipids: sterols(e.g, cholesterol, vitamin D, bile salts, and vitamins A, E, and K)

Examples in patient care:

- Patients are typically advised to be cautious of fat intake, especially those who have undergone a malabsorptive procedure such as the gastric bypass or BPD-DS due to increased risk of dumping syndrome. Patients who have had their gall-bladders removed may also experience dumping syndrome after consuming foods high in concentrated fat.
- Foods high in fat not well tolerated after surgery are pastries or sweets; high-fat dairy products such as cheese, heavy cream, butter, and sour cream; high-fat meat such as red meat or processed red meats like hot dogs, luncheon meat, sausage, or pepperoni; high volume of any type oil at one serving (such as in salad dressings or foods sautéed in excess oil or creamy/rich soups); and fried foods.

31.1.3 Carbohydrates

Energy 5 g/kg

Function Carbohydrates are used primarily to maintain blood glucose concentrations between meals. To ensure readily available supply, all cells store carbohydrates in the easily metabolized glycogen polymer. These are manufactured by plants and are a major source of energy in the diet comprising around half of total calories. Many larger molecules of carbohydrates are not digestible and classified as dietary fiber.

Components

- Monosaccharides (glucose, dextrose, fructose, galactose)
- Disaccharides (sucrose [table sugar], lactose [milk sugar], maltose [malt sugar], oligosaccharides)
- Polysaccharides (amylose, dextrins)
- Dietary fiber and functional fiber

Examples in patient care:

- It is important for patients after weight loss surgery to continue choosing healthy sources of carbohydrates in their diet. Postoperative patients have difficulty tolerating white bread, rice, potatoes, and pasta. Most patients will again be able to include these foods in their diet after some time (typically <3 months).
- High-fiber carbohydrates should be encouraged (4+ grams per serving) including packaged grains, vegetables, non-starchy vegetables prepared without excess oils or fats, fruits, and some dairy foods.
- Foods not recommended for weight loss success are white processed sugar, sweets/candy, sweet baked goods, or sugar-sweetened beverages.
- Patients who have undergone a malabsorptive procedure (Roux-en-Y gastric bypass or biliopancreatic diversion with duodenal switch) are subject to dumping

syndrome. Dumping syndrome is an uncomfortable sensation causing sweating, uncomfortableness, and ultimately rapid digestion of the food from the duodenum to the end of the GI tract leading to urgent diarrhea. This may occur 15–30 min after eating a triggering food or even upward to 1–4 h. This negative reinforcement is often why patients avoid these foods after their weight loss surgery. Foods which are high in concentrated sweets are more likely to trigger this reaction in patients after this surgery for <5 years.

- Fiber
- Dietary fiber: intact plant components that are not digestible by gastrointestinal enzymes
- Functional fiber: nondigestible carbohydrates that have been extracted or manufactured from plants
- Both have been shown to have beneficial physiologic functions in the GI tract and in reducing risk of certain disease states and should be encouraged in a healthy diet to promote weight loss maintenance, healthy cholesterol, and blood pressure.
- There is currently evidence-based research available to support a high-fiber diet in the support of weight loss and weight loss maintenance.
- For every 1000 cal, patients are encouraged to take in <14 g of fiber per day. The recommendation for fiber by the American Heart Association is <25–35 g daily for a 2000 cal diet.
- Patients who do not consume adequate amount of carbohydrate in their diet may be at risk to: fatigue, constipation, slow weight loss, difficulty feeling full, and lethargy.

31.2   Micronutrients

31.2.1 Vitamins

Definition Organic compounds (or class of compounds) distinct from fats, carbohydrates, and proteins. Natural components of foods; usually present in minute amounts. Not synthesized by the body in amounts adequate to meet normal physiologic needs. Specific deficiency syndrome is a result of absence or insufficiency.

Function Essential for normal physiologic function such as maintenance, growth, development, and reproduction.

31.2.1.1   Fat-Soluble Vitamins
- Vitamin A (Retinoids) is found in animal and plant foods. Plants contain carotenoids (most importantly the antioxidant beta-carotene).
  - Function: visual pigments, cell differentiation, and gene regulation.
  - Deficiency: impaired vision, night blindness, or blindness.
  - Sources: egg yolks, vitamin A fortified milk, dark leafy green vegetables such as spinach and kale, and yellow-orange pigmented fruits and vegetables such

as carrots, sweet potatoes, and cantaloupe. Vitamin A is more bioavailable after cooking.
– Toxicity: persistent large doses (over 100 times the recommendation of 200,000 RAE's) may lead to liver disease. Characteristics may be seen in the skin and mucous membranes and lead to dry lips, dry nose and eyes, scaling of the skin, hair loss, fragile nails, headache, nausea, vomiting, and increased risk of hip fractures.
• Vitamin D:
– Function: calcium homeostasis and bone metabolism
– Deficiency: fatigue, hormone imbalance, and osteoporosis
– Sources: sunlight exposure, herring, salmon, fish liver oil, fortified milks and nondairy milks, and fortified cereals
– Toxicity: calcification of the bone, kidney stones, metastatic calcification of soft tissues, hypercalcemia, headache, weakness, nausea, vomiting, constipations, polyuria, and polydipsia
• Vitamin E:
– Function: membrane antioxidant
– Sources: plant oils (sunflower, canola, peanut, corn, olive), nuts (almonds, cashews, mixed nuts), fortified cereal, fruits and vegetables (asparagus, apricots), and grains and grain products such as bran cereal
– Toxicity: decreases ability to use other fat-soluble vitamins
• Vitamin K:
– Function: blood clotting, calcium metabolism
– Sources: green leafy vegetables such as broccoli, cabbage, turnip greens, and dark lettuces. Some dairy, meat, eggs, fruits, and cereals
– Toxicity: hemolytic anemia and severe jaundice

31.2.1.2 Water-Soluble Vitamins
• Vitamin C (Ascorbic acid):
– Function: reductant in hydroxylation in biosynthesis of collagen and carnitine and in the metabolism of drugs and steroids.
– Deficiency: scurvy, impaired wound healing, edema, hemorrhages, weakness in the bone, cartilage and teeth and connective tissues, bleeding gums, lethargy, fatigue, rheumatic pain in legs, muscular atrophy, skin lesions, and various psychological changes.
– Sources: fruits, vegetables, organ meats, citrus fruits, peppers, melon, and strawberries.
– Toxicity: GI disturbances and diarrhea. Excess may also cause renal oxalate stones.
• Vitamin B1 (Thiamine):
– Function: coenzyme for decarboxylations of 2-keto acids and transketolations. Necessary for metabolism and detoxification.
– Deficiency: anorexia, weight loss, cardiac and neurological signs, indigestion, constipation, malaise, "pins and needles" and numbness in legs, increased pulse and palpitations, wet beriberi (edema of legs, face, trunk, and serous cavities; tense calve muscles; distended neck veins; high blood pressure;

decreased urine volume), and dry beriberi (difficulty walking, Wernicke-Korsakoff syndrome, encephalopathy (loss of immediate memory, disorientation, nystagmus, ataxia)).
  - Sources: fortified cereals, yeasts, and liver.
  - Toxicity: 100× greater than recommended levels may lead to headache, convulsions, muscular weakness, cardiac arrhythmia, and allergic reactions. Only in massive doses (1000× greater than nutritional needs) has been seen to suppress the respiratory center causing death.
- Vitamin B2 (Riboflavin):
  - Function: coenzyme in redox reactions of fatty acids and the TCA cycle
  - Deficiency: photophobia, tearing, burning, or itching of eyes; loss of visual acuity; and soreness and burning of lips, mouth, and tongue. Advanced: fissuring of lips; angular stomatitis; greasy eruption of the skin in nasolabial folds, scrotum, or vulva, and purple swollen tongue
  - Sources: green leafy vegetables, fortified cereals, fortified dairy, and nondairy beverages
- Niacin:
  - Function: coenzyme for several dehydrogenases.
  - Deficiency: pellagra (dermatitis, dementia and diarrhea, and death if untreated), muscular weakness, anorexia, indigestion, skin eruptions, tremor, and sore tongue.
  - Sources: peanuts, yeasts, fortified cereals, mushrooms, coffee, lean meats, poultry, and fish.
  - Toxicity: high doses of 1–2 g three times per day increase histamine release causing flushing that can be harmful to those with asthma or peptic ulcer disease. High doses have been also found to be toxic to the liver.
- Vitamin B6 (Pyridoxine):
  - Function: coenzyme in amino acid metabolism
  - Deficiency: weakness, sleeplessness, peripheral neuropathy, cheilosis, glossitis, stomatitis, and impaired cell-mediated immunity
  - Sources: fortified cereals and whole grain products, vegetables, fruits, bananas, beans, nuts, and lean meats
- Biotin:
  - Function: coenzyme for carboxylations
  - Deficiency: alopecia, seborrheic dermatitis, paralysis, and inflammatory bowel disease
  - Sources: peanuts, almonds, soy protein, eggs, yogurt, nonfat milk, and sweet potatoes
- Pantothenic acid:
  - Function: coenzyme in fatty acid metabolism
  - Deficiency: impairment in lipid synthesis and energy production
  - Sources: fortified cereals, nuts, mushrooms, avocado, broccoli, egg yolk, sweet potatoes, lean meats, and skim milk
- Folate:
  - Function: coenzyme in single-carbon metabolism

- Deficiency: impairs biosynthesis of DNA and RNA, thus reducing cell division; Megaloblastic, macrocytic anemia; General weakness, depression, and polyneuropathy.
  - Sources: green leafy vegetables (esp. spinach, broccoli, asparagus), dried beans, mushrooms, potatoes, whole grains, and lean beef.
- B12 (Cobalamin):
  - Function: coenzyme in metabolism of propionate, amino acids, and single-carbon fragments
  - Deficiency: impaired cell division (particularly in the bone marrow and intestinal mucosa) and megaloblastic anemia
  - Sources: fermented foods, nutritional yeast, eggs, cheese, fish, oysters/clams/crab, fortified cereals, liver, kidney, and muscle meats

Examples in patient care:

- It is important for patients to understand the consequences of vitamin deficiency. It is much easier to prevent a deficiency than it is to resolve one.
- After bariatric surgery it is essential for patients to ensure adequate vitamin intake and supplementation as recommended by their bariatric team. Guidelines are set by the American Society of Bariatric and Metabolic Surgery (Table 31.3) [2]. It is important for patients to remain up-to-date on these guidelines for optimal health, weight loss, and repair after surgery.
- It is difficult to meet the body requirements through diet alone since it often takes time to increase caloric intake to more than 1000 cal per day after surgery.
- After malabsorptive procedures the body is unable to process these vitamins through diet alone, and patients require lifelong supplementation:
  - Roux-en-Y vitamin malabsorption: vitamin B12, iron, and calcium
  - Biliopancreatic diversion with duodenal switch: vitamin B12, Iron, calcium, and fat-soluble vitamins A, D, E, and K
- Many patients may come to the office before surgery with preexisting vitamin deficiencies (most commonly vitamin D). Deficiencies should be addressed, and replenishing doses administered as soon as possible before and after surgery.
- After surgery, it is the current recommendation for patients to begin vitamin supplementation when they begin their full liquid diet. Supplements that are best tolerated are liquid, chewable, intramuscular, sublingual, and/or gel capsule.

31.2.2 Minerals

- Definition: Macrominerals and microminerals are essential in absorption, transport, storage, and excretions of many functions in the human body. They are essential for 4–5 % of body weight.
- Function: Macrominerals act as positive ions (cations) where micronutrients act as anions. Minerals exist as components of bones, teeth, phosphoproteins, phospholipids, metalloenzymes, and other metalloproteins such as hemoglobin.

Table 31.3 ASMBS
recommended vitamin
supplementation

Vitamin A	10,000 IU
Vitamin C	120 mg
Vitamin D3	3000–6000 IU
Vitamin E	60 IU
Vitamin K	160 mcg
Thiamin	3 mg
Riboflavin	3.4 mg
Niacin	40 mg
B6	4 mg
Folic acid	400 mcg
B12	1000 mcg
Biotin	60 mcg
Pantothenic acid	20 mg
Calcium	1200–2400 mg
Iron	45–60 mg
Magnesium	400 mg
Zinc	15 mg
Copper	2 mg
Manganese	3.6 mg
Chromium	120 mcg
Molybdenum	90 mcg

- Components:
  - Macrominerals: calcium, magnesium, sodium, potassium, chloride, and sulfur
  - Microminerals: iron, zinc, iodine, selenium, manganese, fluoride, molybdenum, copper, chromium, cobalt, and boron
- Calcium:
  - Function: 99 % is found in bones and teeth. Ionic calcium is essential for ion transport across cell membranes.
  - Sources: dark leafy green vegetables such as kale, broccoli, turnip or mustard greens, tofu, fortified dairy, almonds, blackstrap molasses, bones in canned salmon or sardines, clams, and oysters.
  - Supplementation: for maximum absorption, supplementation should also include vitamin D. After bariatric surgery patients are recommended to supplement their diet with 1200–2400 mg of calcium per day. Calcium in the form of calcium citrate is best absorbed, especially in those with malabsorptive procedures.
  - Toxicity: hypercalcification of soft tissues, bone fractures, and constipation. It may also interfere with absorption of iron, zinc, and manganese.
- Phosphorus:
  - Function: 80 % is found in bones and teeth. Component of every cell and important metabolites in DNA, RNA, ATP, and phospholipids. Also important for Ph regulation
  - Sources: egg yolk, fish, lean meat, and fortified cereal

- Magnesium:
  - Function: 50 % in the bone. Cofactor for many enzymes including those involved in energy production
  - Sources: legumes, fortified cereals, tofu, nuts, green vegetables, milk, and chocolate
- Sulfur:
  - Functions: oxidation reactions as part of thiamin and biotin
  - Sources: legumes, nuts, fish, dairy, and meat
- Iron:
  - Function: 70 % found in hemoglobin, 25 % stored in the spleen, liver, and bone. Component of hemoglobin and myoglobin and important in oxygen transfer
  - Sources: legumes, dark green vegetables, whole or enriched grains, egg yolk, shrimp, oysters, meat, and liver
- Zinc:
  - Function: present in most tissues, particularly the liver, voluntary muscle, and bone. Component of many enzymes and of insulin and zinc and important for nucleic acid metabolism
  - Sources: legumes, wheat bran, shellfish, oysters, herring, and liver
- Copper:
  - Function: found in all body tissues, with the bulk in the brain, liver, heart, and kidney. Integral part of DNA and RNA
  - Sources: cherries, legumes, chocolate, nuts, whole grains, liver, shellfish, kidney, poultry, and oysters
- Iodine:
  - Function: constituent of thyroid hormone and related compounds synthesized by the thyroid gland, control of reactions involving cellular energy
  - Sources: sea vegetables, seafood, and iodized salt
- Manganese:
  - Function: highest concentration is in the bone and also in the pituitary, liver, gastrointestinal tissue, and pancreas; high in mitochondria of liver cells; and constituent of essential enzyme systems
  - Sources: legumes, nuts, blueberries, beet greens, and whole grains
- Fluoride:
  - Function: essential for the mineralization of bones and teeth
  - Sources: drinking water, tea, coffee, spinach, gelatin, and onion
- Molybdenum:
  - Function: constituent of essential enzymes and flavoproteins
  - Sources: legumes, cereal grains, and dark leafy greens
- Cobalt:
  - Function: constituent of vitamin B12. Essential for the normal function of all cells specifically bone marrow, GI systems, and nervous systems
  - Sources: liver, kidney, oysters, clams, poultry, and milk
- Selenium:
  - Function: involved in fat metabolism, acts as antioxidant, and cooperates with vitamin E

- Sources: grains, onions, milk, and meat
- Chromium:
  - Function: associated with glucose metabolism
  - Sources: whole grain cereals, brewer's yeast, drinking water, and clams

31.2.3 Water

- Patients are advised to consume at least 48–64 oz water or clear liquids for optimum hydration after surgery. It is recommended to also monitor hydration by observing urine color output. If color is dark or amber with a strong odor, they are dehydrated.
- Drinking adequate fluids is typically the biggest challenge after surgery since they are only able to safely tolerate ½ ounce every half hour at the hospital.
- Patients should be coached into increasing the ½ ounce every ½ hour interval until goal rate of 3 oz every 30 min is achieved.
- Drinking can feel like a "full-time job" to some patients. It is critical to be patient with them during this time and to encourage their success. Even at 3 ounces every half hour, once they get home, they are recommended to sip 4–6 ounces at a time every hour. This can become tiresome and for most patients unusual. There is a learning curve to obtain adequate fluids after surgery due to reasons such as inflammation, soreness, and the sensitivity to the new sensation of a smaller stomach pouch.
- Dehydration is the number one reason for readmission after surgery.
- If it is gathered, a patient is experiencing dehydrations (dark urine, dizzy, dizzy upon standing, constipation, dry mouth, headaches, fatigue). They should hydrate immediately, and if it is too difficult, they should go to the nearest emergency department for IV fluids.
- If a patient becomes dehydrated, it can be helpful to use a beverage that contains electrolytes, especially if they are experiencing headaches or vomiting (e.g., ORAGIN electrolyte replacement, coconut water, low-sodium vegetable juice, or other sugar-free sports drinks).

31.2.4 Other Nutritional Tidbits

- Antioxidants: molecules such as some vitamins (C and E) that block action of activated oxygen molecules (free radicals) that can damage cells
- Phytochemicals: nonnutritive compounds in plants thought to influence the process of tumorigenesis
- Alcohol after bariatric surgery
  - A patient may reach their peak blood alcohol content within 10 min of an alcoholic beverage because of alteration of gastric anatomy. It is recommended to abstain from alcohol consumption for the first 6 months to 1 year after bariatric surgery for safety.

For nutrition review questions, please see the next two chapters.

References

1. Mahan K, Escott-Stump S, Raymond J, Krause M (2012) Krause's food & the nutrition care process. Elsevier/Saunders, St. Louis
2. American Society for Metabolic and Bariatric Surgery. Integrated Health Nutritional Guidelines – American Society for Metabolic and Bariatric Surgery; 2016. [Online]

Alyssa Luning, Cheri Leahy, and Lisa Harasymczuk

Upon initial nutrition consultation with a patient, a bariatric registered dietitian will review their current dietary patterns, habits, and typical intake. This assessment will help to better understand where the patient currently is before establishing dietary goals. From the assessment, the dietitian will begin to meet the patient where they are to begin implementing behavior change. It is important to establish changes the patient will have to make before surgery, so they have more of an opportunity to practice adapting. Establishing goals relating to diet, dietary habits, physical activity, and resolving biochemical complications is very important for the individual alongside of patient nutrition education on the preop diet, vitamins and minerals after surgery, common complaints, meal planning, goal setting, and diet stages after surgery.

Dietary habit changes may include the following: begin scheduling meals at regular intervals, discontinue meal skipping, begin multivitamins, and increase fruits and vegetables, lean proteins, whole grains, legumes, low-fat dairy, and possibly protein shakes. As needed, it is recommended for them to begin eliminate or reduce unhealthy snack foods such as packaged sweets, crackers/chips, fried foods, fast food, sugar-sweetened beverages, carbonated beverages, alcoholic beverages, and soda. Other dietary changes include not drinking with meals, avoiding caffeine 2 weeks before surgery, taking 20–30 min per meal time, chewing well at meals, and preparing for their 2-week preoperative diet. It is important for the patient to express understanding of the importance of changing their diets and dietary habits as needed to promote weight loss success.

It is helpful for recent lab work to be taken before surgery. A general review of current vitamin and glucose levels as well as a lipid panel can work as a prompter

A. Luning, RDN • C. Leahy, RDN (✉)
Kennedy Health Alliance, 2201 Chapel Ave W #100, Cherry Hill, NJ 08002, USA
e-mail: a.luning@kennedyhealth.org; cherileahyrd@gmail.com

L. Harasymczuk, DO
Department of General Surgery, Rowan University, Stratford, NJ, USA

© Springer International Publishing Switzerland 2017
A. Loveitt et al (eds), *Passing the Certified Bariatric Nurses Exam*,
DOI 10.1007/978-3-319-41703-5_32

for specific dietary changes as well as any supplementation if needed. If a dietary or supplemental intervention is needed, prompt action before surgery will improve overall patient health and weight loss afterward. Without proper review before surgery, a patient may be at an increased risk of worsening iron and or vitamin D deficiency. These deficiencies may impair the healing process, and may have a negative impact on successful weight loss.

The most common preoperative medical nutrition therapy interventions deal with elevated blood glucose and or A1c, elevated cholesterol, elevated low-density lipoprotein (LDL) cholesterol, low high-density lipoprotein (HDL) cholesterol, elevated triglycerides, and supplementation of vitamin D and/or iron if a patient is found to have a deficiency [1].

During preoperative nutrition education, patients should be educated on the 2-week preop diet. This program has been found to significantly decrease risks and complications before, during, and after their surgery. This works by decreasing the liver's storage of carbohydrates and fatty acids which shrinks the size of the liver by 50–60 % making it easier for the surgical team to access the stomach. Up to 50 % of patients have nonalcoholic steatohepatitis or fatty liver. This is significantly decreased within the 2 weeks of the diet. The diet itself is low in fat and carbohydrates and most often includes the use of high-protein meal replacement shakes. The specifics of the 2-week diet vary from practice to practice depending on the surgeon and dietitians. With proper compliance, patients also experience a loss in weight, about 5–10 pounds that helps to shrink the abdominal cavity and provides an additional confidence boost [2].

Upon compliance to dietary changes, vitamin supplementation, dietary behaviors, physical activity changes, and the use of the 2-week preop diet, patients are more confident, prepared, ready, and rearing to undergo their life-changing operation. Depending on the individual's choice of surgical team, dietitian, and their health insurance, their preoperative education may vary in length and quality. Always check with the patient to see what they already know or if they have any further questions whenever an opportunity arises. There are so many things changing in their lives at once, and it can seem overwhelming at times. Always be considerate to the individual who is about to begin the first day of the rest of their lives after surgery.

32.1 Nutritional Follow-Up

After bariatric surgery, it is very valuable for the patient to follow up with his or her registered dietitian in the office within 5–7 days. This is helpful to monitor their tolerance of fluids, volume of fluids, and any complications they may be experiencing soon after surgery such as dizziness, light-headedness, nausea, constipation, heartburn, or gas. As the patient begins to increase volume of fluids he or she is able to tolerate per sitting, the dietitian or health professional will establish a reasonable time to begin to advance his or her diet. After that appointment, nutritional follow-up with a registered dietitian is recommended by most practices to continue monitoring the success and give additional support to the patient. Some offices may have a set structure of an appointment every 3 months post-op in the first year and then annually, and some offices may offer little pre-contemplated structure. It is ultimately up to the patient how much nutritional follow-up they include in their care after surgery.

There is significant research to show a higher success rate in weight loss and weight loss maintenance with those who do follow with a registered dietitian compared with those who do not [1, 2]. After the surgery, the hard work is typically just beginning. Follow-up may help ground the patient by providing a place of accountability as well as a place to check in on biochemical status, vitamins, and or complications such as persistent vomiting, constipation, nausea, heartburn, slow weight loss, or weight loss plateaus. Working with a registered dietitian, patients are able to stay on track with their meal planning, exercise, and healthy lifestyle habits as they explore their new lives after weight loss surgery. Registered dietitians are trained to remain up to date and are licensed. They are educated in core healthcare sciences as well as food science, food systems, public health, psychology, and counseling skills and sometimes more depending in their area of special interest or expertise making them preferable providers for medical nutrition therapy.

Review Questions

1. How much daily protein is recommended following bariatric surgery?

   A. 60–80 g for women and 80–100 g for men
   B. 20–40 g for women and 40–60 g for men
   C. 40–60 g for both women and men
   D. 80–100 g for both women and men

2. What are complete proteins?

   A. They complete the bariatric diet.
   B. They contain all of the protein needed for the bariatric diet.
   C. They include all amino acids.
   D. They include only the essential amino acids.

3. Which procedure is more likely to cause dumping syndrome postoperatively?

   A. Sleeve gastrectomy
   B. Roux-en-Y gastric bypass
   C. Gastric banding

4. Which of these foods is most likely to cause dumping syndrome?

   A. Processed sugars
   B. Steamed vegetables
   C. Bread
   D. Fresh fruits

5. When should patients start their vitamin supplementation postoperatively?

   A. Postoperative day 0
   B. Postoperative day 1
   C. When they start their bariatric clear liquid diet
   D. When they start their bariatric full liquid diet

6. What is the number one reason for readmission after surgery?

   A. Pain
   B. Nausea
   C. Dehydration
   D. Diarrhea

7. How many fluid ounces should be consumed daily postoperatively?

   A. 28–44
   B. 48–64
   C. 68–84
   D. 88–104

8. How long should a patient wait to drink alcohol postoperatively?

   A. 7–10 days
   B. 14–21 days
   C. 1–3 months
   D. 6 months–1 year

9. For maximum absorption, calcium supplementation should be paired with vitamin D supplementation, true or false?

   A. True
   B. False

10. Deficiency of this vitamin causes dermatitis, dementia, and diarrhea.

   A. Vitamin B1
   B. Vitamin B2
   C. Niacin
   D. Vitamin B6

Answers

1. The answer is A. Generally it is recommended protein requirements after bariatric surgery are 60–80 g for women and 80–100 g for men. It is important to appreciate that patients may have difficulty meeting these goals initially and should focus on staying hydrated.
2. The answer is C. Complete proteins contain all amino acids.
3. The answer is B. Dumping syndrome results after the Roux-en-Y when a food bolus enters the small intestine after bypassing the stomach. This

causes a rapid shift in fluids and can lead to bloating and abdominal pain. This is a much less frequent problem after sleeve gastrectomy or gastric band.

4. The answer is *A*. Dumping syndrome, as described above, can occur with any food but most commonly occurs after eating processed foods (sugars, sweets, soda, cakes). To prevent dumping syndrome, patients are encouraged to eat small frequent meals and avoid drinking half an hour before and after eating.

5. The answer is *D*. Patients should start taking their vitamin supplementation when they start their full liquid (stage II) diet, typically around post-op day 5.

6. The answer is *C*. The number one reason for readmission after bariatric surgery is dehydration. Patients should be counseled pre- and postoperatively to help avoid this. They are encouraged to sip liquids "like it's their job" to maintain hydration. An easy gauge is for patients to drink until their urine is clear.

7. The answer is *B*. Patients are encouraged to drink at least 48–64 fl oz per day postoperatively.

8. The answer is *D*. Patients should wait 6 months to 1 year before introducing social alcohol back into their diet. At this point they should be accustomed to how their body reacts and responds after their surgery. It is important to council them that absorption of alcohol may be much more rapid than before their surgery and they should continue to be very cautious.

9. The answer is *A*. Calcium absorption is paired with vitamin D in the gut. Any calcium supplementation is best paired with vitamin D to assure adequate absorption.

10. The answer is *C*. Niacin deficiency is classically described as leading to the three "D's" diarrhea, dermatitis, and dementia.

References

1. Mahan K, Escott-Stump S, Raymond J, Krause M (2012) Krause's food & the nutrition care process. Elsevier/Saunders, St. Louis
2. American Society for Metabolic and Bariatric Surgery. Integrated Health Nutritional Guidelines – American Society for Metabolic and Bariatric Surgery. 2016. [Online]

Follow-Up and Dietary Progression After Bariatric Surgery

33

Nidhi Khanna, Cheri Leahy, and Alyssa Luning

The decision to undergo bariatric surgery is a lifelong commitment. Close postoperative follow-up is essential to the success of the operation and to ensure patients maintain weight loss.

The follow-up will vary by surgeon, but a typical schedule after laparoscopic adjustable gastric band (LAGB) is 2 weeks and 6 weeks postoperatively. After this, patients may follow up every 4–6 weeks for 1 year and then every 6 months [1, 2]. For laparoscopic Roux-en-Y gastric bypass (LRYGB) and laparoscopic sleeve gastrectomy (LSG) patients, follow-up is more frequent. This starts at 2 weeks post-op and then months 1, 3, 6, 9, 12, 18, and 24. After this patients may follow up every year [2].

Diet progression, again, varies by surgeon and patient. A clear liquid diet (stage 1) is started within 24 h after the operation and continued while an inpatient. Dietary goals should be reinforced by a nutritionist prior to discharge. After discharge, a full liquid (stage 2) diet is started by postoperative day 5, soft (stage 3) is started by two weeks post-op, and solid foods (stage 4) are reintroduced at approximately 1 month (Table 33.1). Dehydration is a common reason for readmission, and it should be stressed to the patient to take in 64 fluid ounces of liquids a day. Patients are advised to avoid concentrated sweets, carbonation, and use of straws. Protein goals are 1.5 g/kg ideal body weight per day, but a minimum of 60 g per day is recommended [2].

Although exceptions may be made in select patients (such as those whose musculoskeletal pain is limiting their mobility), anti-inflammatory medications like ibuprofen and aspirin are avoided because of the increased risk of ulcer formation. Furthermore they are advised to abstain from smoking, especially those who

N. Khanna, DO
Department of General Surgery, Rowan University, Stratford, NJ, USA
e-mail: khannani@rowan.edu

C. Leahy, RDN (✉) • A. Luning, RDN
Kennedy Health Alliance, 2201 Chapel Ave W #100, Cherry Hill, NJ 08002, USA
e-mail: cherileahyrd@gmail.com; a.luning@kennedyhealth.org

© Springer International Publishing Switzerland 2017
A. Loveitt et al (eds), *Passing the Certified Bariatric Nurses Exam*,
DOI 10.1007/978-3-319-41703-5_33

Table 33.1 Recommended dietary progression after bariatric surgery

Diet advancement	Allowed foods	Duration
Stage 1 – clear	Clear liquids Examples: protein powder added to any clear liquids, amino acid complex mixed in water, and clear broth or stock (chicken, beef, veal, vegetable mushroom, miso) Water, unsweetened decaf iced tea, diluted fruit juices, decaffeinated tea/coffee, true lemon beverages, sugar-free Jell-O Coconut water and sugar-free popsicles	Day 1–4 (During hospital stay and at home until able to reach goal rate of 3 oz water every 30 min)
Stage 2 – full	Full liquids Examples: protein drink, fat-free (skim) milk, unsweetened nondairy milk, blended split pea, bean, vegetable, or lentil soup, sugar-free/low-sugar, fat-free/low-fat, or fat-free Greek-style yogurt. Sugar-free pudding thinned with fat-free milk. Unsweetened applesauce, unsweetened pureed fruits, smooth/creamy hot cereal	Day 5–15 Patients may begin to take their bariatric multivitamins and other supplements
Stage 3 – soft	Soft "mush-able" foods Examples: lentils or split peas, black beans, cannellini beans, red kidney beans, black beans, fat-free refried beans, tofu, banana, peaches, or pears (if canned, no added sugar), sweet potato, cooked carrots, cauliflower, broccoli, string beans, winter squash Low-fat cottage cheese Low-fat or fat-free ricotta cheese Soft scrambled egg or egg whites Soft well-cooked (Crock-Pot or ground meat) chicken or turkey, Fish (tuna, salmon, crab meat, tilapia)	Day 15–30
Stage 4 – solid	Regular texture bariatric diet OK to introduce raw vegetables such as salad greens, crunchy fruits such as apples, and nuts/seeds	Day 31-3 mo
Beyond	Solid, low fat/low sugar, high fiber Typically, OK to decrease high-protein diet and increase dietary fiber per patient goals	Day 90+

underwent LRYGB due to risk of marginal ulcer formation at the gastrojejunal anastomosis [2].

Activity is limited to ambulation in the first few postoperative weeks. Patients can then slowly increase exercise regimens to incorporate cardiovascular and weight training routines to facilitate weight loss.

Follow-up with a general medical physician as well as subspecialties such as endocrine, cardiology, etc., is also important. Post-op bariatric patients will need reevaluation of chronic medical illnesses and adjustments of respective medications [1, 2].

Review Questions

1. Which of the following are important factors to stress to bariatric patients in the immediate postoperative period?

   A. Incentive spirometry
   B. Ambulation
   C. Hydration
   D. Avoidance of concentrated sweets
   E. All of the above

2. Which of the following has not been shown to be associated with more weight loss in post-bariatric surgery patients?

   A. Attending support groups
   B. Joining an exercise program
   C. Eating large meals less frequently
   D. Adherence to follow-up visits

3. Three weeks after a RNYGB, your post-op bariatric patient is hospitalized for nausea and vomiting. After inquiring the patient, you learn the patient has been eating chicken and vegetables three times a day with fruit for snacks. What is the correct diet 3 weeks after LRYGB?

   A. Clear liquids
   B. Fulls liquids
   C. Pureed foods
   D. Solid foods
   E. None of the above

Answers

1. The answer is *E*. Postoperative bariatric patients are at high risk for venous thromboembolism (VTE), atelectasis and pneumonia, and dehydration. Therefore, it is important for all the members of the bariatric team to encourage patients to ambulate (B) in order to prevent VTE. In addition, the use of incentive spirometry (A) and deep breathing exercises is essential in preventing patients from having pulmonary complications. Lastly, hydration (C) with liquids that DO NOT contain concentrated sweets (D) is important to prevent dehydration and unnecessary caloric intake.

2. The answer is *C*. Results from multiple studies and recommendations from the ASMBS (American society for metabolic and bariatric surgery) concur on factors that lead to more weight loss in post-op bariatric patients. Attending support groups (A), joining an exercise program (B), and adherence to follow-up visits (D) have all shown trends toward better weight loss outcomes. Eating smaller meals three times a day is advised in addition to maintaining higher protein intake and eliminating concentrated sweets.

3. The answer is *C*. After RNYGB and LSG, patients are started on a bariatric stage 1 diet or clear liquids (A) and continued on this for 2 weeks. From weeks 2 to 4, patients are on full liquids (B). From 1 month to 3 months, the patient is on pureed foods (C), and after 3 months they are advanced to solid foods (D).

References

1. Favretti F et al (2002) Patient management after LAP-BAND placement. Am J Surg 184:38s–41s
2. Mechanick J et al (2013) Clinical practice guidelines for the perioperative nutritional, metabolic, and nonsurgical support of the bariatric surgery patient. Surg Obes Relat Dis 9:159–191

Additional Review Questions

1. Which of the following laparoscopic procedures is a purely restrictive weight loss surgery?

   A. Sleeve gastrectomy
   B. Roux-en-Y gastric bypass
   C. Laparoscopic gastric band
   D. Jejunal-ileal bypass
   E. None of the above

   The answer is *C*. Weight loss surgery can be divided into two categories, restrictive and malabsorptive procedures. Choice C, gastric band does not remove a portion of the stomach or alter normal anatomy or physiology. This is why it is only a restrictive procedure. Ingested food is limited which allows for more frequent meal intake, less caloric intake, and weight loss. In contrast to this, choices A, B, and D are all categorized as having at least some malabsorptive properties.

2. All of the following are the components of the gastric banding device *Except*:

   A. Subcutaneous port
   B. Port tubing
   C. Inflatable band
   D. Balloon implant
   E. None of the above

   The answer is *D*. Subcutaneous port (A), port tubing (B), and inflatable band (C) are all parts of the gastric banding device. The inflatable band is placed around the upper portion of the stomach and is connected to the band tubing. The tubing is brought out through the anterior abdominal wall and tunneled in the subcutaneous tissues and attached to the port. The port is sutured under the skin in the subcutaneous tissues. Choice D, the balloon implant is not part of the banding apparatus.

© Springer International Publishing Switzerland 2017
A. Loveitt et al. (eds.), *Passing the Certified Bariatric Nurses Exam*,
DOI 10.1007/978-3-319-41703-5

3. Which of the following is an appropriate patient for weight loss surgery?

   A. 55-year-old healthy female with a BMI of 28
   B. 25-year-old male with a BMI of 30, history of diabetes, and no attempt at exercising or dietary modification
   C. 40-year-old male with hypertension and sleep apnea, BMI 37
   D. 37-year-old female with a BMI of 40 who has missed several preoperative appointments
   E. 60-year-old female with a BMI of 33, history of alcohol dependence and diabetes

   The answer is *B*. It is important to know how to choose the appropriate patient for bariatric surgery. A BMI of 30 with comorbid conditions such as diabetes, obstructive sleep apnea, and hypertension or a BMI of 40 with no associated conditions are general criteria for weight loss surgery. In addition to this, patients must be compliant (D), must undergo a psychiatric and nutritional workup, and have tried diet and exercise modifications to lose weight (B). Patients with drug or alcohol dependence are also excluded from undergoing surgery (E).

4. Which of the following are important factors to stress to bariatric patients in the immediate post-operative period?

   A. Incentive spirometry
   B. Ambulation
   C. Hydration
   D. Avoidance of concentrated sweets
   E. All of the above

   The answer is *E*. Post-operative bariatric patients are at high risk for venous thromboembolism (VTE), atelectasis and pneumonia, and dehydration. Therefore, it is important for the all members of the bariatric team to encourage patients to ambulate (B) in order to prevent VTE. In addition, the use of incentive spirometry (A) and deep breathing exercises are essential in preventing patients from having pulmonary complications. Lastly, hydration (C) with liquids that *do not* contain concentrated sweets (D) is important to prevent dehydration and unnecessary caloric intake.

5. Which of the following has *not* been shown to be associated with more weight loss in post-bariatric surgery patients?

   A. Attending support groups
   B. Joining an exercise program
   C. Eating large meals less frequently
   D. Adherence to follow-up visits

   The answer is *C*. Results from multiple studies and recommendations from the ASMBS concur on factors that lead to more weight loss in post-op bariatric patients. Attending support groups (A), joining an exercise program (B), and adherence to follow-up visits (D) have all shown trends toward better weight loss outcomes. Eating smaller meals three times a day is advised in addition to maintaining higher protein intake and eliminating concentrated sweets.

6. Which one of the following is not an indication to get gastric bypass surgery?

   A. Morbid obesity with a BMI greater than 40
   B. BMI greater than 35 with two comorbidities
   C. To lose weight due to multiple attempts at trying to lose weight and being unable to do so
   D. To boost one's self-esteem

   The answer is *D*. While a boost in self-esteem is a welcomed effect of weight loss surgery, it, in itself, is not an indication. For a patient to qualify, they must have a BMI >40 or >35 with a comorbid condition. Most physicians and insurances also require documentation that the patient has had failed weight loss attempts in the past.

7. Which one of the following is not typically related to tachycardia?

   A. Bleeding
   B. Dehydration
   C. Urinary retention
   D. Pain
   E. Anxiety

   The answer is *C*. Tachycardia, especially if sustained >120 bpm, is a concerning sign in the post-operative bariatric patient. It can result from bleeding or a leak. Additional causes to consider include pain, anxiety, and dehydration. Urinary retention does not typically result in tachycardia, although if it is left untreated long enough, the patient may develop severe suprapubic pain.

8. Which of the following is not a long-term complication of bypass?

   A. Anastomotic stricture
   B. Internal hernia
   C. Vitamin deficiencies
   D. Wound infection
   E. Cholelithiasis (gallstones)

   The answer is *D*. Wound infections occur in the immediate post-op period and can typically be treated with local drainage and control. Anastomotic stricture could potentially occur immediately due to technical error but often occurs as a long-term complication. Internal hernias, vitamin deficiencies, and cholelithiasis all occur in the late post-operative period.

9. A relatively healthy 46-year-old male, who is a long-distance truck driver, with a BMI of 41, arrives to the recovery room after a gastric bypass and abdominal hernia repair surgery. The patient is placed on his CPAP with oxygen at that time. Once his pain and respirations are stabilized, he is transferred to the surgical unit. He remains on O2 2 L nasal cannula and his vital signs are in the normal range. His nurse admits him to the unit, completing the history and physical assessment, and he answers all the questions. In a few hours, after the patient has rested, the nurse observes that the patient has shallow breaths and he is perspiring. His vital signs are only slightly changed except that his respirations

are shallow at 40 (tachypnea), the pulse ox is 83 %, and he states that "it hurts to take a deep breath." The patient is seen by the surgical team and a STAT ABG is drawn. His PaO2 is 85 mmHg (hypoxemia). The first and most frequently seen pulmonary complication is:

A. Obstructive sleep apnea (OSA)
B. Chest pain
C. Respiratory alkalosis
D. Atelectasis

The answer is *D*. Atelectasis occurs as a result of the effects of anesthesia, seen by the absence of sigh breaths which help to reinflate the lungs, especially in cases with longer surgery time. Also the depressive side effects of pain relievers or narcotics as well as the feeling of incisional pain can decrease tidal volumes. Basically, one or more areas of the lung collapse or do not inflate properly which decreases oxygen saturation. This is the first and most frequent pulmonary complication! There is no evidence of cardiology involvement in this scenario. The patient could possibly have respiratory acidosis but it is not mentioned.

10. Tests that detect this complication include all *Except*:

A. ABG
B. Pulse ox
C. EKG
D. Chest x-ray

The answer is *C*. EKG is necessary for a cardiology diagnosis, but the other three tests help diagnose pulmonary complications.

11. What could have prevented this complication?

A. Frequent additional doses of pain medication
B. Early ambulation
C. Elevation of the patient's legs while in bed
D. Administering an IV fluid bolus

The answer is *B*. Early ambulation can prevent or minimize atelectasis because walking will increase the lung's tidal volume and minimize pressure of the diaphragm on the lungs. Multiple or frequent doses of narcotics can depress respirations. Elevation of legs and additional IV fluids do not improve the lung capacity.

12. The nurse discovers that the patient's pain level is a "10 out of 10." After administering morphine 1 mg IV for pain, what other measures should be taken?

A. Teach the patient how to use the incentive spirometer 10 times every hour and to splint his abdomen to cough.
B. Elevate his chest and head while in bed.
C. Utilize the patient's CPAP and supplemental oxygen when he is resting.
D. Once the patient's pulse ox is equal to or above 92 %, have him sit up in the chair.
E. All the above.

The answer is *E*. Upon arrival to the unit, the clinical nurse should instruct the patient on how to use the incentive spirometer and have him demonstrate its use. The patient should have his head elevated to allow improved respirations and tidal volume. Because the patient arrived to the unit in a slightly sedated state, the nurse should have placed the patient on O2 and his CPAP. Ambulating or sitting up in the chair will improve his respiratory status and possibly prevent pulmonary complications.

13. A long-term consequence of OSA, obesity, sleep deprivation, hypoxemia, and hypoventilation is:

A. Left-sided heart failure
B. Pickwickian syndrome
C. Low CO2 level
D. Hyperventilation

The answer is *B*. Pickwickian syndrome, better known as obesity-hypoventilation syndrome, includes right-sided heart failure, hypertrophy, swollen legs, elevated CO2 levels, and hypoventilation. Patients with these symptoms are often treated with progestational agents and the use of a CPAP during sleep times.

14. Contraindications to bariatric surgery include all of these *Except*:

A. Irreversable pulmonary disease
B. Unstable or advanced cardiac disease
C. Sleep apnea
D. Inflammatory bowel disease or intestinal motility disorders

The answer is *C*. Bariatric patients require pulmonary clearance before surgery due to many having diagnosed or not diagnosed OSA. A decrease in the pharyngeal area, from an increase in fat tissue in the pharynx lateral pharyngeal walls, results in OSA. With significant weight loss after bariatric surgery, the patient may no longer need a CPAP! The other three choices are ALL contraindications to bariatric surgery.

15. The patient is discharged after a 48 h hospital stay, and he plans to return to his truck driving job within 5 days, as he needs the income. What medication will the surgeon most likely prescribe for this patient during the discharge process?

A. Ibuprofen 600 mg oral every 6 h around the clock
B. Albuterol inhaler—one puff every 4 h as needed for SOB
C. Dilaudid 2 mg oral every 4 h around the clock
D. Lovenox 40 mg SQ to the abdomen daily in the morning for 14 days

The answer is *D*. The patient sits almost the entire day while driving long distances in his truck. His risk for DVT is greater due to immobility and lack of exercise. The physician will encourage this patient to make frequent stops to stretch his legs and ambulate. Ibuprofen is an NSAID which is not recommended post surgery due to its risk for stomach ulcers. Dilaudid would not be prescribed ATC because it is a narcotic with a side effect of drowsiness, so this patient cannot drive while taking medication. However, he could have Dilaudid as a PRN prescription as long as he knows not to drive while taking it for pain. For minor aches and pain, Tylenol is a better choice. Albuterol inhaler is a good medication but not a priority, and the patient will most likely follow up with a pulmonologist as an outpatient.

16. What is the first and second most common cause of death to the bariatric patient?

   A. Myocardial infarction and pulmonary embolism
   B. Pulmonary embolism and deep vein thrombosis
   C. Pulmonary hypertension and pneumonia
   D. Pulmonary embolism and anastomotic/intestinal leak

   The answer is *D*. A blood clot in the lung and a leak of gastrointestinal contents are both dreaded complications of bariatric surgery with high mortality rates. While the other complications listed above can occur, they are not as frequent causes of death.

17. What are some late complications of bariatric surgery?

   A. MI, GERD, respiratory distress, pneumonia
   B. Pulmonary embolism, wound infection, bleeding of suture lines
   C. Bowel obstruction, gallstones, dumping syndrome
   D. GERD, pulmonary embolism, food intolerance

   The answer is *C*. Bowel obstruction could develop later, but not initially. Due to a rapid weight loss, the patient has an increase risk of gallstones developing. Most patients at some time will experience dumping syndrome.

18. Common gastric bypass surgery risks include:

   A. Bleeding, anastomotic leaks, infection
   B. Anastomotic stenosis, ulceration
   C. Incisional hernia and nutrient/calorie malnutrition
   D. All the above

   The answer is *D*. All of the above are risks related to the gastric bypass which the patient should be counseled on preoperatively.

19. All of the below are factors that may affect medication dosages in obese patients *Except*:

   A. Increased fatty tissue
   B. Increased total body water
   C. Increased blood volume
   D. Elevated cardiac output
   E. Increased renal blood flow and glomerular infiltration rate

   The answer is *B*. Obese patients actually have a decrease in total body water.

20. There are higher rates of obesity in:

   A. Women and children
   B. Men and ethnic groups

C. Women and ethnic groups
D. African Americans and men

The answer is C. Besides women, the ethnic groups also include African Americans, Caucasians, and Hispanics.

21. What is the fastest growing obesity trend in the USA?

A. BMI > or equal to 40
B. BMI > or equal to 50
C. BMI > 35–39.9
D. BMI > 25–29.9

The answer is B. Nine million people in the USA are severely obese with a BMI equal to or above 50.

22. Obesity and surgery are two cumulative risk factors for DVT. What are some additional risks?

A. Age > 35 years and a smoker
B. BMI > 25 and taking estrogen or HRT
C. Immobility and a smoker
D. Female and BMI > 30

The answer is C. The average age of > 45 years, immobility, heart and respiratory failure, history of venous stasis disease, smoking, male, elevated BMI, and being on prescribed estrogen or hormone replacement therapy are cumulative risk factors for DVT.

23. What health history increases the risk of a DVT the most?

A. MI
B. Smoking
C. Diabetes
D. OSA

The answer is B, smoking.

24. Bariatric surgery patients are a risk for DVT/PE complications. Thrombosis prophylaxis strategies may include:

A. Aspirin 325 mg daily starting post-op day 1
B. Vena cava filters for all bariatric patients
C. Continuous IV heparin drip immediately after surgery
D. Low dose unfractionated heparin administer every 6 h SQ

The answer is D. Also, early ambulation and the use of sequential compression sleeves would be additional prophylaxis strategies. While some surgeons may select to place inferior vena cava (IVC) filters in some patients, placing them in all patients is not a typical strategy.

25. What comorbid condition may increase the risk for infection?

A. OSA
B. BMI > 40

C. Diabetes

D. GERD

The answer is *C*. Diabetes increases risk for poor wound healing and infection.

26. A syndrome caused by injury to the skeletal muscle in which intracellular muscle contents are released into the circulation is:

A. Tubular necrosis

B. Hypovolemia

C. MI

D. Rhabdomyolysis

The answer is *D*. The risk increases with patients who are especially in the higher BMI levels. Rhabdomyolysis can result in renal damage and failure treatment includes avoidance of nephrotoxic agents and aggressive intravenous fluid resuscitation.

27. The lab test result for a patient with suspected rhabdomyolysis will show a:

A. Low CPK

B. Rise in CPK

C. High lactate level

D. Low potassium level

The answer is *B*. The rise in the CPK level could indicate an early sign of rhabdomyolysis; thus, urine output should be measured and the patient should be receiving adequate hydration.

28. The study of choice for patients with increased bariatric post-operative pain is:

A. Abdominal survey ultrasound

B. EGD

C. Upper GI

D. CT scan

The answer is *C*. The UGI can detect gastroesophageal reflux disease (GERD) or esophagitis changes, can detect gastric pouch dilatation and stomach widening, can show ulcers, and is the best test to detect gastric leaks. In reality, a CT scan is often the first test ordered in the emergency department but would not be the study of choice.

29. What is the treatment for port infection following laparoscopic adjustable band?

A. Wear an abdominal binder

B. Irrigation and debridement of the wound

C. Antibiotics and possible removal of the port if the infection does not clear

D. Dressing changes to the infection site two times per day

The answer is *C*. Antibiotics is the best choice for treatment for a gastric band port infection. Removal would occur if the infection does not clear.

30. Nearly 85 % of bypass surgery patients experience a specific gastrointestinal complication called:

A. GERD
B. Constipation
C. Gastric ulcer
D. Dumping syndrome

The answer is *D*. It is very common that most patients will at some time experience this unpleasant issue when eating too many sweets or carbohydrates.

31. Early dumping syndrome occurs 30–60 min after eating including symptoms of:

A. Fever, cramping
B. Chills, nausea
C. Sweating, tachycardia
D. Constipation, fever

The answer is *C*. Early dumping syndrome results from a rapid influx of a hyperosmotic load into the gut and can lead to sweating and tachycardia. Other symptoms could possibly include lightheadedness, nausea, diarrhea, tachycardia, palpitations, cramping, and audible bowel sounds.

32. When does late dumping syndrome occur? What are the symptoms?

A. 1–2 h and constipation
B. 1–3 h and hyperglycemic episodes
C. 1–3 h and hypoglycemic episodes
D. 30 min and sweating

The answer is *C*. Late dumping syndrome occurs 1–3 h after eating from the rapid influx of insulin that results from early dumping. Symptoms include: hypoglycemic episodes, sweating, shakiness, hunger, loss of concentration, and fainting.

33. A 55-year-old female with a BMI of 48 has gastric bypass and hernia surgery. Post-operatively, she constantly complains of pain and numbness in her left forearm. What complication is she most likely experiencing?

A. MI
B. Frequent BPs taken on the left arm
C. Ulnar nerve compression/injury
D. Muscle fatigue

The answer is *C*. During surgery, the most common injury, ulnar (elbow) nerve injury, results from compression or straining of the nerve due to pushing on the arm, trying to be closer to the patient, or excessive positioning by trying to move the arm out of the way.

34. Due to the weight of the bariatric patient, it is important that the hospital equipment should include:

    A. Bariatric ceiling lift to transfer or reposition patients when necessary
    B. The use of pillows or wedges as cushions to protect pressure points
    C. Restraints to prevent falls
    D. Expanded capacity (EC) equipment, marked with a weight capacity rating
    E. A,B, and D

    The answer is *E*. Depending on the BMI and health capacity of the patient, a ceiling lift should be available to patients who cannot transfer themselves. Also any caregiver who has to lift >35 pounds of weight should require assistive equipment for that patient. Pillows and wedges can be used as cushions to protect pressure points and limb positioning during surgery is crucial to prevent injuries. Some helpful equipment in the OR may include expanding tables and extra arm and foot boards. High weight capacity on all equipment, such as beds, chairs, and stretchers, is a considered standard practice to accommodate the patient's weight and sometimes their visitors.

35. Other considerations for this female patient may include:

    A. Gowns that are readily available to fit comfortably
    B. Toilets that are wall based with large seats
    C. Stretcher that holds 300 pound limit
    D. Standard hospital bed

    The answer is *A*. Gowns, adjustable ID bracelets, floor-based toilets, 1000 pound capacity stretchers, and expanding capacity beds would be useful and less stigmatizing if the supplies were readily available without embarrassing the patient.

36. One of the most common health complications during rapid weight loss is:

    A. Incisional hernias
    B. Urinary tract infections
    C. Stomach fistulas
    D. Cholelithiasis (gallstones)

    The answer is *D*. Gallstones are known to occur with rapid weight loss.

37. Another similar health complication due to calcium abnormalities and inadequate hydration is:

    A. Hypercalcemia
    B. Dumping syndrome
    C. Kidney stones
    D. Anastomotic leak

    The answer is *C*. Gallstones are the most common complication of calcium deposition with rapid weight loss, but kidney stones can develop under such circumstances as well, especially if the patient is not well hydrated on a daily basis. A concentrated urine over time increases the risk for developing kidney stones.

38. The hormones produced or secreted in the intestinal tract to regulate appetite are listed below *Except*:

    A. Cholecystokinin
    B. Ghrelin
    C. Leptin
    D. Peptide yy

    The answer is *C*. Although all hormones listed above play a role in appetite, leptin is actually secreted by white adipose tissue in direct proportions of total body fat. Cholecystokinin is secreted by the duodenum and jejunum. Ghrelin is secreted by the fundus (stomach). Peptide yy is released by the descending colon and rectum.

39. Commonly seen cardiac comorbid conditions of bariatric patients may include:

    A. Murmurs, hypotension
    B. Hypertension, abnormal lipid levels
    C. Hyponatremia, gallops
    D. Abnormal lipid levels and hypotension

    The answer is *B*. Murmurs or gallops, structural or functional changes in the heart, CAD, MI, heart failure, valvular disease, hypertension, sodium retention, and abnormal lipid levels are all common cardiac comorbid conditions.

40. Common skin findings in obese patients include:

    A. Acne and ecchymosis
    B. Hirsutism and fungal infections
    C. Cellulitis and acne
    D. Psoriasis and cellulitis

    The answer is *B*. Common skin disorders are fungal infections, cellulitis, stasis ulcers, hirsutism possibly from polycystic ovary syndrome or Cushing's syndrome, and ecchymosis possibly due to Cushing's syndrome.

41. Common metabolic complications of obesity could include:

    A. HTN, Type II DM, hypercoagulopathy
    B. Dyslipidemia, pancreatitis
    C. Gallstones, OSA
    D. Polycystic ovarian syndrome, nonalcoholic fatty liver disease
    E. All the above

    The answer is *E*. The epidemic of obesity has brought with it a drastic rise in all of the above listed conditions.

42. Women with obesity may see all of these symptoms *Except*:

    A. Hirsutism
    B. Infertility
    C. Irregular menses
    D. Low levels of estradiol

The answer is *D*. One could see elevated levels of estradiol which is produced in relation to the amount of adipose (fat) tissue.

43. Surgeons will council childbearing-aged female patients whose:

    A. Weight loss increases their chances for C-sections in the future.
    B. Preterm births are common with bariatric surgery patients.
    C. They must wait 12–18 months post surgery before becoming pregnant.
    D. Risk of cancers increases with weight loss.

    The answer is *C*. Surgery candidates should avoid pregnancy preoperatively and also 12–18 months post-operatively both because of the increased risk for VTE with pregnancy and perioperative nutritional deficiencies. It has been found that breast, endometrial, and cervical cancers are at a higher risk with obesity, not with weight loss. Both A and B hold no evidence.

44. In order to reduce the risk for post-operative thromboembolic phenomena, the surgeon will council female patients to:

    A. Continue estrogen therapy.
    B. Discontinue 1 cycle or month of oral contraceptives in premenopausal women prior to surgery.
    C. Discontinue hormone replacement therapy 1 week prior to surgery for post-menopausal women.
    D. Discontinue estrogen therapy after surgery for 3 weeks.

    The answer is *B*. The doctor will discontinue estrogen therapy. Postmenopausal women are to stop HRT 3 weeks prior to surgery. Oral contraceptives are typically held for 1 month after surgery, and patients are asked to use alternative forms of birth control. Choice D does not apply.

45. A 40-year-old obese female that is considering bariatric surgery presents to her physician with neurological symptoms of tinnitus, visual problems, and headaches. What could be her diagnosis?

    A. Multiple sclerosis
    B. Stress headaches
    C. Brain tumor
    D. Pseudotumor cerebri

    The answer is *D*. Obese women of childbearing age can present with pseudotumor cerebri. Symptoms include headache behind the eyes, tinnitus, blurred vision, brief episodes of blindness, light flashes, and neck, shoulder, or back pain. The symptoms mimic a brain tumor, but there is no tumor. Instead, there is an excess amount of cerebral spinal fluid in the skull, causing intracranial hypertension.

46. A post-operative gastric bypass patient from 3 weeks ago has symptoms of distress, tachycardia, nausea, vomiting, and epigastric pain. This patient could have:

A. GERD
B. Esophagitis
C. Gastric remnant distention
D. UTI

The answer is *C*. The roux-en-Y gastric bypass leaves the stomach intact to drain through the biliopancreatic limb and eventually through the jejunal-jejunal anastomosis. If this outflow is obstructed, it can result in the above symptoms. An early cause could be due to hematoma (obstructing blood clot) in the remnant, which may require surgery. Decompression may possibly be used if the remnant is dilated with gastric secretions.

47. A 60-day post-operative laparoscopic band was deflated on a male patient who was losing weight too quickly and he was appearing malnourished. He is at a higher risk for what metabolic complication in the next few days?

A. Refeeding syndrome
B. GERD
C. Hypoglycemia
D. Increase levels of thiamine

The answer is *A*. An individual with a rapid weight loss can be susceptible for RS within days of starting to feed. This patient will most likely develop a fluid and electrolyte imbalance. He may also have neurological, pulmonary, cardiac, neuromuscular, or blood complications.